Effect of Long-Term Insomnia on Mental Health

Effect of Long-Term Insomnia on Mental Health

Guest Editor

Aleksandra M. Rogowska

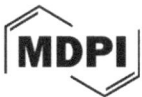

Basel • Beijing • Wuhan • Barcelona • Belgrade • Novi Sad • Cluj • Manchester

Guest Editor
Aleksandra M. Rogowska
Institute of Psychology
University of Opole
Opole
Poland

Editorial Office
MDPI AG
Grosspeteranlage 5
4052 Basel, Switzerland

This is a reprint of the Special Issue, published open access by the journal *Journal of Clinical Medicine* (ISSN 2077-0383), freely accessible at: https://www.mdpi.com/journal/jcm/special_issues/0HLCOFD228.

For citation purposes, cite each article independently as indicated on the article page online and as indicated below:

Lastname, A.A.; Lastname, B.B. Article Title. *Journal Name* **Year**, *Volume Number*, Page Range.

ISBN 978-3-7258-4375-6 (Hbk)
ISBN 978-3-7258-4376-3 (PDF)
https://doi.org/10.3390/books978-3-7258-4376-3

© 2025 by the authors. Articles in this book are Open Access and distributed under the Creative Commons Attribution (CC BY) license. The book as a whole is distributed by MDPI under the terms and conditions of the Creative Commons Attribution-NonCommercial-NoDerivs (CC BY-NC-ND) license (https://creativecommons.org/licenses/by-nc-nd/4.0/).

Contents

Zosia Goossens, Thomas Bilterys, Eveline Van Looveren, Anneleen Malfliet, Mira Meeus, Lieven Danneels, et al.
The Role of Anxiety and Depression in Shaping the Sleep–Pain Connection in Patients with Nonspecific Chronic Spinal Pain and Comorbid Insomnia: A Cross-Sectional Analysis
Reprinted from: *J. Clin. Med.* **2024**, *13*, 1452, https://doi.org/10.3390/jcm13051452 1

Omar Gammoh, Abdelrahim Alqudah, Esam Qnais, Alaa A. A. Aljabali, Ammena Y. Binsaleh and Sireen Abdul Rahim Shilbayeh
Are Sleep Aids Associated with the Severity of Attention Deficit Hyperactivity Disorder Symptoms in Adults Screened for Insomnia? A Cross-Sectional Study
Reprinted from: *J. Clin. Med.* **2024**, *13*, 1682, https://doi.org/10.3390/jcm13061682 15

Adonis Sfera, Kyle A. Thomas, Isaac A. Ogunjale, Nyla Jafri and Peter G. Bota
Insomnia in Forensic Detainees: Is Salience Network the Common Pathway for Sleep, Neuropsychiatric, and Neurodegenerative Disorders?
Reprinted from: *J. Clin. Med.* **2024**, *13*, 1691, https://doi.org/10.3390/jcm13061691 25

Angelia M. Holland-Winkler, Daniel R. Greene and Tiffany J. Oberther
The Cyclical Battle of Insomnia and Mental Health Impairment in Firefighters: A Narrative Review
Reprinted from: *J. Clin. Med.* **2024**, *13*, 2169, https://doi.org/10.3390/jcm13082169 44

Jessica Dagani, Chiara Buizza, Herald Cela, Giulio Sbravati, Giuseppe Rainieri and Alberto Ghilardi
The Interplay of Sleep Quality, Mental Health, and Sociodemographic and Clinical Factors among Italian College Freshmen
Reprinted from: *J. Clin. Med.* **2024**, *13*, 2626, https://doi.org/10.3390/jcm13092626 62

Tahani K. Alshammari, Aleksandra M. Rogowska, Anan M. Alobaid, Noor W. Alharthi, Awatif B. Albaker and Musaad A. Alshammari
Examining Anxiety and Insomnia in Internship Students and Their Association with Internet Gaming Disorder
Reprinted from: *J. Clin. Med.* **2024**, *13*, 4054, https://doi.org/10.3390/jcm13144054 72

Carlos Roncero, José Bravo-Grande, Diego Remón-Gallo, Pilar Andrés-Olivera, Candela Payo-Rodríguez, Alicia Fernández-Parra, et al.
The Relevance of Insomnia Among Healthcare Workers: A Post-Pandemic COVID-19 Analysis
Reprinted from: *J. Clin. Med.* **2025**, *14*, 1663, https://doi.org/10.3390/jcm14051663 89

Omar Gammoh, Abdelrahim Alqudah, Mariam Al-Ameri, Bilal Sayaheen, Mervat Alsous, Deniz Al-Tawalbeh, et al.
Prevalence and Risk Factors of Mobile Screen Dependence in Arab Women Screened with Psychological Stress: A Cross-Talk with Demographics and Insomnia
Reprinted from: *J. Clin. Med.* **2025**, *14*, 1463, https://doi.org/10.3390/jcm14051463 100

Wendemi Sawadogo, Anuli Njoku and Joy Jegede
Insomnia Symptoms, Mental Health Diagnosis, Mental Health Care Utilization, and Perceived Barriers in U.S. Males and Females
Reprinted from: *J. Clin. Med.* **2025**, *14*, 2989, https://doi.org/10.3390/jcm14092989 109

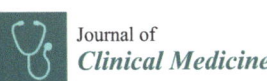

Article

The Role of Anxiety and Depression in Shaping the Sleep–Pain Connection in Patients with Nonspecific Chronic Spinal Pain and Comorbid Insomnia: A Cross-Sectional Analysis

Zosia Goossens [1,2,*], Thomas Bilterys [1,3,4,5], Eveline Van Looveren [1,6], Anneleen Malfliet [1,3,7], Mira Meeus [1,8], Lieven Danneels [6], Kelly Ickmans [1,3,9], Barbara Cagnie [6], Aurore Roland [2,7,10], Maarten Moens [11,12,13], Jo Nijs [1,3], Liesbet De Baets [1,3,*,†] and Olivier Mairesse [2,10,14,15,†]

[1] Pain in Motion Research Group (PAIN), Department of Physiotherapy, Human Physiology and Anatomy, Faculty of Physical Education & Physiotherapy, Vrije Universiteit Brussel, Laarbeeklaan 103, 1090 Brussels, Belgium; thomas.bilterys@vub.be (T.B.); eveline.van.looveren@vub.be (E.V.L.); anneleen.malfliet@vub.be (A.M.); mira.meeus@uantwerpen.be (M.M.); kelly.ickmans@vub.be (K.I.); jo.nijs@vub.be (J.N.)
[2] Brain, Body and Cognition, Department of Psychology, Faculty of Psychology and Educational Sciences, Vrije Universiteit Brussel, 1050 Brussels, Belgium; aurore.roland@vub.be (A.R.); olivier.mairesse@vub.be (O.M.)
[3] Department of Physical Medicine and Physiotherapy, Universitair Ziekenhuis Brussel, Laarbeeklaan 101, 1090 Brussels, Belgium
[4] Institute of Advanced Study, University of Warwick, Coventry CV4 7AL, UK
[5] Department of Psychology, University of Warwick, Coventry CV4 7AL, UK
[6] Department of Rehabilitation Sciences and Physiotherapy, Faculty of Medicine and Health Sciences, Ghent University, Campus Heymans, 9000 Ghent, Belgium; lieven.danneels@ugent.be (L.D.); barbara.cagnie@ugent.be (B.C.)
[7] Research Foundation-Flanders (FWO), 1000 Brussels, Belgium
[8] MOVANT Research Group, Department of Rehabilitation Sciences and Physiotherapy, Faculty of Medicine and Health Sciences, University of Antwerp, 2000 Antwerpen, Belgium
[9] Movement & Nutrition for Health & Performance Research Group (MOVE), Department of Movement and Sport Sciences, Faculty of Physical Education and Physiotherapy, Vrije Universiteit Brussel, Pleinlaan 2, 1050 Brussels, Belgium
[10] Brussels University Consultation Center, Department of Psychology, Faculty of Psychology and Educational Sciences, Vrije Universiteit Brussel, 1090 Brussels, Belgium
[11] Department of Neurosurgery, Universitair Ziekenhuis Brussel, 1090 Brussels, Belgium; maarten.ta.moens@vub.be
[12] Department of Radiology, Universitair Ziekenhuis Brussel, 1090 Brussels, Belgium
[13] Center for Neurosciences (C4N), Vrije Universiteit Brussel (VUB), 1090 Brussels, Belgium
[14] Vital Signs and PERformance Monitoring (VIPER), LIFE Department, Royal Military Academy, 1000 Brussels, Belgium
[15] Laboratoire de Psychologie Médicale et Addictologie, CHU/UVC Brugmann, 1020 Brussels, Belgium
* Correspondence: zosia.goossens@vub.be (Z.G.); liesbet.de.baets@vub.be (L.D.B.); Tel.: +02-629-20-10 (Z.G.)
† These authors contributed equally to this work.

Abstract: (1) Background: This exploratory study aims to explore the relationship between nonspecific chronic spinal pain (nCSP) and insomnia symptoms, by examining the interconnections, strengths, and directional dependence of the symptoms. In addition, we aim to identify the key symptoms of the nCSP–insomnia relationship and shed light on the bidirectional nature of this relationship. (2) Methods: This study is a secondary analysis of the baseline data (cross-sectional) from a randomized controlled trial, which examined the added value of Cognitive Behavioral Therapy for Insomnia (CBT-I) combined with cognition-targeted exercise therapy, conducted in collaboration with the Universiteit Gent and Vrije Universiteit Brussel (Belgium). One hundred and twenty-three nCSP patients with comorbid insomnia were recruited through the participating hospitals, advertisements, announcements in local newspapers, pharmacies, publications from support groups, and primary care. To explore the interconnections and directionality between symptoms and the strengths of the relationships, we estimated a regularized Gaussian graphical model and a directed acyclic graph. (3) Results: We found only one direct, but weak, link between sleep and pain, namely, between average pain and difficulties maintaining sleep. (4) Conclusions: Despite the lack of strong direct links between sleep and pain, pain and sleep seem to be indirectly linked via anxiety and depression symptoms, acting as presumable mediators in the network of nCSP and comorbid insomnia. Furthermore, feeling slowed down and fatigue emerged as terminal nodes, implying their role as consequences of the network.

Keywords: chronic pain; low back pain; network analysis

1. Introduction

Nonspecific chronic spinal pain (nCSP) and insomnia are two common and debilitating conditions that significantly impact an individual's quality of life [1–3]. Furthermore, nCSP is associated with absenteeism leading to high socioeconomic consequences [4]. nCSP, encompassing chronic low back pain, chronic neck pain, and failed back surgery syndrome, is a widespread condition and is defined as chronic if the pain occurs on most days and lasts for at least three months [1,4]. Insomnia, on the other hand, is the most common sleep disorder which manifests as a subjective complaint in initiating, maintaining sleep, and/or waking up sooner than desired. In addition, at least one daytime impairment must be present (e.g., concentration difficulties, mood swings, malaise, sleepiness, or fatigue). Insomnia becomes chronic when it persists for at least three months and occurs at least three nights a week [1,5–7]. Insomnia is the most common comorbidity reported among persons with nCSP, and previous research indicates a strong, bidirectional association between nCSP and insomnia [1,7].

Although a reciprocal relationship between pain and sleep seems well accepted [8–11], multiple studies consider disturbed sleep a better predictor of pain than vice versa [2,8–12]. The contribution of insomnia to the development or amplification of pain is suggested to lie in alterations in pain processing and hyperalgesic responses [8,9]. However, the complexity of the relationship between pain and sleep leaves many remaining questions, such as the potential underlying factors of the direction and strength of the association [12]. These potential factors could lie in prevalent complaints of both persons with insomnia and chronic pain, such as fatigue, symptoms of anxiety, and symptoms of depression [13–15]. Although the domain of fatigue and nCSP is less studied, reduction of fatigue is one of the patient-determined success criteria for the treatment of nCSP [16]. On the other hand, symptoms of anxiety and depression are suggested to at least partially mediate the relationship between pain and sleep. Persons with insomnia might be more vulnerable to symptoms of anxiety and depression, as improvement in these symptoms improves sleep disturbance. However, improvements in anxiety and depression do not often predict changes in pain [8,10,12,17,18].

In order to deepen our understanding of the complexity of the relationship between sleep and pain, network approaches should be considered. Such a network approach considers symptoms as constitutive components of a disorder, actively influencing and maintaining each other through direct causal interactions. It uses graph theory to represent symptoms as nodes and their interrelations as edges, which can be visualized and analyzed [19,20]. A Gaussian graphical model (GGM) represents conditional independence associations in an undirected graph. Meanwhile, a cross-sectional directed acyclic graph (DAG) reveals directional dependencies, indicating a stronger influence of one node on another. Integrating these models allows for inferring potential causal relations among nodes [21,22]. Hence, this approach allows us to move beyond the traditional latent variable models and gain a deeper understanding of the dynamic interactions between symptoms of nCSP, insomnia, anxiety, depression, and fatigue [20,23–27].

Given the exploratory opportunities of the network approach, this study aims to provide further insights into the sleep–pain relationship by examining the interconnections, strengths, and directional dependence of symptoms of nCSP, insomnia, anxiety, depression, and fatigue. In addition, we aim to identify the key symptoms in the network. These insights could offer promising avenues for enhancing the overall non-pharmacological management and quality of life for persons suffering both conditions.

2. Materials and Methods

2.1. Participants

This study is a secondary analysis of the baseline data (cross-sectional) from a randomized controlled trial, which examined the added value of incorporating Cognitive Behavioral Therapy for Insomnia (CBT-I) into the current best physical therapy treatment for nonspecific chronic spinal pain (nCSP). The full study protocol was registered at clinicaltrials.gov (no. NCT03482856) [3]. This study was a multicenter, cross-sectional study, performed by researchers from Vrije Universiteit Brussel and Ghent University. Participants were recruited through the universities and their corresponding hospitals, advertisements, and announcements in local newspapers, pharmacies, publications from patient support groups, and primary care [3]. The selection criteria can be found in Table 1. In total, 123 patients with CSP and comorbid insomnia were included in the study. The definition of insomnia included self-reported sleep difficulties, defined as >30 min of wake during the night [including sleep latency, wake after sleep onset, early morning awakenings, or a combination] for >3 days/week for >6 months, which cause distress or impairment in daytime functioning (despite having adequate opportunity and circumstances to sleep) in the absence of intrinsic sleep disorders and shift work. Polysomnography was used for the identification of intrinsic sleep disorders. Obstructive sleep apnea was defined as an apnea–hypopnea index over 15, and periodic leg movement disorder as a periodic limb movement index over 15. The scoring of these indices followed the American Academy of Sleep Medicine Manual for Scoring of Sleep and Associated Events guidelines [28]. This study was approved by the ethics committee of the Ghent University Hospital (2018/0277) and the University Hospital Brussels (2018/077).

Table 1. Selection criteria.

Inclusion	Exclusion
Aged between 18 and 65 years	Body Mass Index > 30, since this study used the baseline data of an RCT investigating an intervention
Native Dutch speaker	Being diagnosed with chronic widespread pain syndrome (e.g., fibromyalgia and chronic fatigue syndrome)
Experiencing nonspecific spinal pain for at least 3 months, at least 3 days/week, including chronic low back pain (CLBP), failed back surgery syndrome (i.e., surgery more than 3 years ago and anatomically successful surgery without symptom disappearance), and chronic traumatic and nontraumatic neck pain	Thoracic pain in the absence of neck or low back pain Neuropathic pain
Experiencing insomnia: self-reported sleep difficulties defined as >30 min of wake during the night [including sleep latency, wake after sleep onset, early morning awakenings, or a combination] for >3 days/week for >6 months, which cause distress or impairment in daytime functioning (despite having adequate opportunity and circumstances to sleep) in the absence of intrinsic sleep disorders and shift work	History of specific spinal surgery (i.e., surgery for spinal stenosis) to ensure the exclusion of degenerative (joint) diseases.
Not undertaking exercise (>3 metabolic equivalents) 3 days before the assessments	Severe underlying sleep pathology (identified through polysomnography), This includes sleep apnea (AHI > 15) and periodic limb movement disorder (>15/h).
Refraining from analgesics, caffeine, alcohol, or nicotine for 48 h before the assessments, since this study used the baseline data of an RCT investigating an intervention	Shift workers

Table 1. Cont.

Inclusion	Exclusion
Willing to participate in therapy sessions and not allowed to continue any other therapies (i.e., other physical therapy treatments, acupuncture, osteopathy, etc.), except for usual medication; and not having received any form of pain neuroscience education or sleep training before	Being pregnant or being a parent within one year post partum
Not starting new treatments or medication and continuing their usual care 6 weeks before and during study participation (to obtain a steady state)	Presence of a current clinical depression diagnosed by a doctor
	Suffering from any specific medical condition possibly related to their pain (e.g., neuropathic pain, a history of neck or back surgery in the past 3 years, osteoporotic vertebral fractures, and rheumatologic diseases)
	People living more than 50 km away from the treatment location were excluded to avoid dropout because of practical considerations.

2.2. Sociodemographic Information

Age, sex, dominant pain problem (neck pain or low back pain), pain duration, and BMI were collected.

2.3. Questionnaires

Participants filled out several questionnaires to assess self-reported sleep such as the Insomnia Severity Index (ISI) [29] and the Pittsburgh Sleep Quality Index (PSQI) [30], as the third edition of the *International Classification of Sleep Disorders* (ICSD-3) and the *International Classification of Diseases*, 11th Revision (ICD-11), recommend a diagnosis of insomnia purely based on subjective complaints [31–33]. Fatigue and sleepiness were assessed using the Brugmann Fatigue Scale (BFS) [34] and Epworth Sleepiness Scale (ESS) [35]. Beliefs and attitudes around sleep were assessed using the Dysfunctional Beliefs and Attitudes About Sleep Scale (DBAS) [36]. Pain-related outcomes were captured by the Brief Pain Inventory (BPI) [37] and Central Sensitization Inventory (CSI) [38]. Mental and physical functioning was assessed using the Short Form Health Survey-36 (SF-36) [39]. Additionally, symptoms of anxiety and depression were evaluated using the Hospital Anxiety and Depression Scale (HADS) [40]. The outcomes of items in these questionnaires were used to select nodes for the pain–sleep network.

An item selection of the above-mentioned questionnaires was carried out as the data were collected in the context of a RCT, and a small number of nodes are recommended to increase power, decrease conceptual overlap, and ensure more stable networks. We used a theoretical approach to review all items and selected nodes based on the hypothesis of representing unique constructs [41–43]. By employing nodes based on an item level, we avoided topological overlap, which would arise when two nearly similar symptoms would be included and lead to inflated edges in the network [44,45]. An overview of the selected items per questionnaire is provided in Table 2.

Table 2. Item selection.

Number	Variable Name	Question	Answer Options
1	ISI1	Difficulty falling asleep?	None/mild/moderate/severe/very severe
2	ISI2	Difficulty staying asleep?	None/mild/moderate/severe/very severe
3	ISI3	Problems waking up too early?	None/mild/moderate/severe/very severe
4	ISI4	How satisfied/dissatisfied are you with your current sleep pattern?	Very satisfied/satisfied/neutral/dissatisfied/very dissatisfied
5	ISI7	To what extent do you consider your sleep problem to interfere with your daily functioning (e.g., daytime fatigue, mood, ability to function at work, daily chores, concentration, memory, mood, etc.) currently?	Not at all interfering/a little/somewhat/much/very much interfering
6	BPIav	Please rate your pain by marking the box beside the number that best describes your pain on average.	0 (No pain)–10 (pain as bad as you can imagine)
7	SF21	How much bodily pain have you had during the past 4 weeks?	Not at all/slightly/moderately/severe/very severe
8	SF22	During the past 4 weeks, how much did pain interfere with your normal work (including both work outside the home and housework)?	Not at all/a little bit/moderately/quite a bit/extremely
9	HADS1	In the past week I have been feeling tense or 'wound up'	0 (Not at all)–3 (most of the time)
10	HADS5	In the past week I had worrying thoughts go through my mind	0 (Only occasionally)–3 (a great deal of the time)
11	HADS8	In the past week I have been feeling as if I am slowed down	0 (Not at all)–3 (nearly all the time)
12	HADS11	In the past week I have been looking forward with enjoyment to things	0 (As much as I ever did)–3 (hardly at all)
13	SF31	Did you feel tired?	All of the time/most of the time/some of the time/a little bit of the time/none of the time

Legend: ISI, Insomnia Severity Index; BPI, Brief Pain Inventory; SF, Short Form Health Survey-36; HADS, Hospital Anxiety and Depression Scale. Numbers represent the items in the survey.

To ensure that the selected items were scored in the same direction (e.g., a high score equals a poor outcome) and to reduce bias, we standardized and transformed the selected items [46].

2.4. Statistical Analysis

Data were analyzed with R software (version 2023.06.0+421, available at https://r-project.org and version 2022.02.4+500 to run Rgraphviz accessed on 5 September 2023). To estimate, visualize, and measure the stability of the networks, the packages *networktools*, *bootnet*, *ggplot2*, *bnlearn*, *Rgraphviz*, and *qgraph* were used [24,45]. First, we estimated a regularized Gaussian graphical model (GGM) using the graphical least absolute shrinkage and selection operator (gLASSO) combined with the Extended Bayesian Information Criterion (EBIC) [45]. Additionally, the cormethod was set to cor_auto (polychoric correlations), the hyperparameter γ (gamma) was set to 0.5, the number of lambda values tested was 100, the network was not thresholded, and the ratio of lowest lambda value compared to maximal lambda was set to 0.01 [41,45]. The additional analysis included centrality measures (strength and expected influence) with the R package *qgraph*, edge-weights accuracy using bootstrapped confidence intervals (1000 bootstraps), the stability of the edges and centrality measures, the significance of differences between edges within the network using the bootstrapped difference test, bridge symptoms, and bridge centrality and stability measures [24]. Due to some unexpected negative edges, an additional network was estimated using Spearman correlations to compare with the Gaussian graphical model. Two very different networks would indicate an untrustworthy estimation of the polychoric correlations [25]. Second, we estimated a directed acyclic graph (DAG) using a Bayesian hill-climbing algorithm with 50 restarts and 100 perturbations [43,47]. There were no specifications for the edges, meaning that all possible edges were allowed in the network [48].

3. Results

3.1. Descriptives

The entire sample was included in the network analyses, which comprised 123 persons with nCSP and comorbid insomnia. The mean pain duration of the participants was 90.03 months (SD = 96.08). The participants' age ranged from 21 to 61 years (M_{age} = 40.36, SD_{age} = 11.06), and the sample included 82 females (67%; M_{age} = 39.46, SD_{age} = 10.99) and 41 males (33%; M_{age} = 42.15, SD_{age} = 11.09). The mean BMI was 23.33 (SD_{BMI} = 3.14).

3.2. Regularized Gaussian Graphical Model

3.2.1. Description

Figure 1 depicts the regularized GGM of nCSP patients with comorbid insomnia and consists of 13 nodes, divided into four clusters: sleep, pain, fatigue, and anxiety and depression symptoms. The network was sparse due to the gLASSO estimation. The network comprised 28 non-zero edges out of 78 possible edges, which were mainly positive. The mean weight of these edges was rather low (M = 0.05).

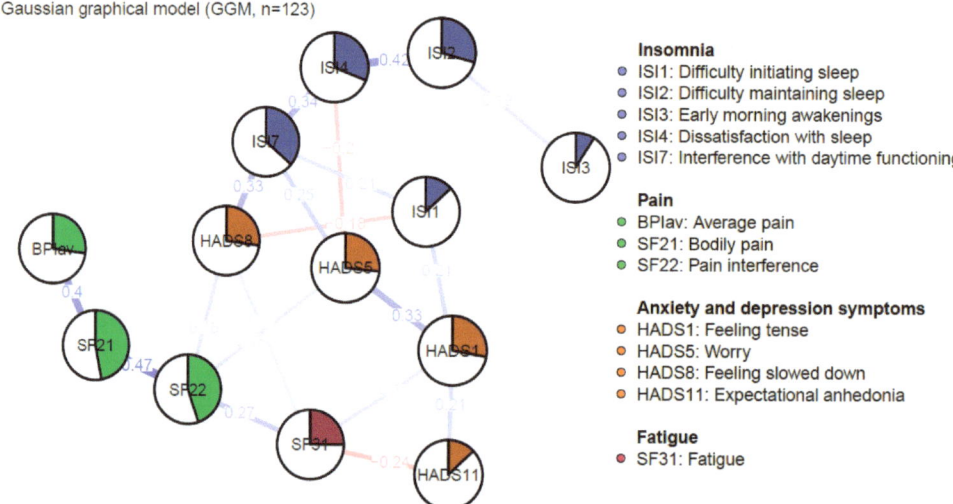

Figure 1. Regularized Gaussian graphical model of pain, insomnia, and affective symptoms: undirected conditional independence associations. The edge's thickness denotes the magnitude of the pairwise association between nodes (i.e., regularized partial correlations, with a maximum set to 1). Positive associations are visualized with blue edges, while red edges represent negative associations. The pies in the nodes reflect predictability, meaning the proportion of the explained variance of the node by all other nodes in the network.

3.2.2. Stability

The stability of a network refers to the consistency and resistance to change. Thus, a stable network entails a set of edges, directions, and centrality measures that are unlikely to change considerably [48]. Based on the benchmarks of Epskamp et al. (2018), the stability of the expected influence centrality of the Gaussian graphical model was acceptable, but not ideal (expected influence CS-C = 0.29) [24]. The confidence intervals resulting from the non-parametric bootstrap analysis were rather broad and overlapping. Therefore, the network and the centrality measure should be interpreted with care. Additionally, due to the poor stability of the bridge and strength centrality, they were not interpreted in the present study (bridge strength CS-C = 0.05; bridge expected influence CS-C = 0.05; strength CS-C = 0.05) (see Supplementary Materials).

3.2.3. Predictability

The measure of predictability is the proportion of variance of a node explained by all other nodes in the network, and ranges between zero (the node is not predictable based on other nodes in the network) and one (other nodes of the network can predict the node at hand perfectly). The mean predictability was 0.27. The node "Bodily pain" was the most determined by all other nodes with 46% variance explained (SF21, R^2 = 0.46). Other relatively predictable constructs were "Pain interference" (SF22, R^2 = 0.44), and "Interference with daytime functioning" (ISI7, R^2 = 0.36).

3.2.4. Edges

Edges represent regularized partial correlations between constructs. The strongest edges appeared between nodes of the same cluster. In the pain cluster, the strongest edge emerged between "Bodily pain" and "Pain interference" (SF21–SF22, r_p = 0.47). In the sleep cluster, the strongest edge appeared between "Difficulty maintaining sleep" and "Dissatisfaction with sleep" (ISI2–ISI4, r_p = 0.42). In the anxiety and depression symptoms cluster, the strongest edge appeared between "Tension" and "Worry" (HADS1–HADS5, r_p = 0.33). Other relatively strong edges emerged between "Feeling slowed down" and "Interference with daytime functioning" (HADS8–ISI7, r_p = 0.33), and "Bodily pain" and "Average pain" (SF21–BPIav, r_p = 0.4). However, according to the edge-weights difference test, these edges are not significantly stronger when compared to each other (see Supplementary Materials). Furthermore, there are no direct, or at best weak, edges between the sleep and pain clusters. The clusters seem to be indirectly connected through the anxiety and depression symptoms. Out of these nodes, both sleep and pain variables showed the strongest connection with "Feeling slowed down". Nevertheless, sleep constructs were more strongly connected in comparison to pain constructs (ISI7–HADS8, r_p = 0.33; SF22–HADS8, r_p = 0.18).

Due to some unexpected negative edges, a Spearman correlation was calculated to evaluate the presence of an artificially induced negative partial correlation via a common effect between "Dissatisfaction with sleep" and "Worry" (ISI4–HADS5), "Feeling slowed down" and "Difficulty initiating sleep" (HADS8–ISI1), and "Fatigue" and "Expectational anhedonia" (SF31–HADS11) [25]. This resulted in a non-significant difference, which means that an artificially induced edge was observed in the regularized partial correlation network between the nodes "Dissatisfaction with sleep" and "Worry" (ISI4–HADS5, p = 0.42), "Feeling slowed down" and "Difficulty initiating sleep" (HADS8–ISI1, p = 0.61), and "Fatigue" and "Expectational anhedonia" (SF31–HADS11, p = 0.31) (see Supplementary Materials).

3.2.5. Centrality Measures

Expected influence is the sum of the value of its connections with other nodes in the network and assesses the node's influence on its neighboring nodes [21]. As seen in Figure 2, the highest expected influence was found in "Pain interference" (SF22, expected influence = 1.60). Relatively high expected influence was also found in "Tension" (HADS1, expected influence = 1.30), "Interference with daytime functioning" (ISI7, expected influence = 1.12), and "Bodily pain" (SF21, expected influence = 0.70). The centrality difference test indicated that only the nodes with the highest centrality values differed from those with the lowest centrality values (see Supplementary Materials).

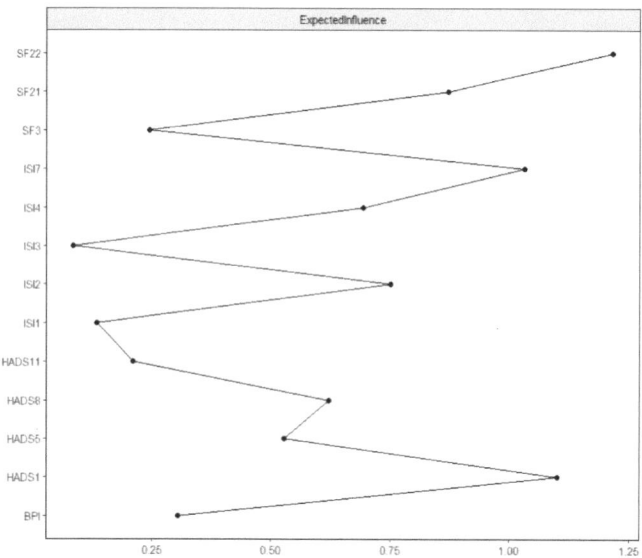

Figure 2. GGM centrality plot: Expected influence. The values on the x-axis represent the unstandardized scores of the centrality measure.

3.3. Directed Acyclic Graph

Cross-sectional DAGs reveal directional dependence relations, where the presence of one node more strongly implies the presence of another than vice versa. This enables us to suggest the underlying causal relations between nodes when used in combination with a GGM [21,22]. Figure 3 shows the DAG with the 13 nodes of the pain and sleep network, where only edges greater than 0.25 are depicted. There are several notable features. First, the DAG revealed a chain of constructs dependent on the parent nodes "Expectational anhedonia" and "Tension". Both showed equal probability of predicting each other, regardless of the direction. While "Tension" appeared to equally predict "Difficulties initiating sleep" and vice versa, it did show a probability of direction to "Worry" greater than 0.5. Therefore, the occurrence of worry is more likely dependent on the presence of tension than vice versa. Second, pain and sleep nodes did not directly predict each other, except for "Average pain" which directly predicted "Difficulty maintaining sleep". Lastly, "Fatigue" and "Feeling slowed down" are terminal nodes in the DAG, with edges from "Pain interference" and "Interference with daytime functioning". These terminal nodes showed equal probabilities of direction between each other.

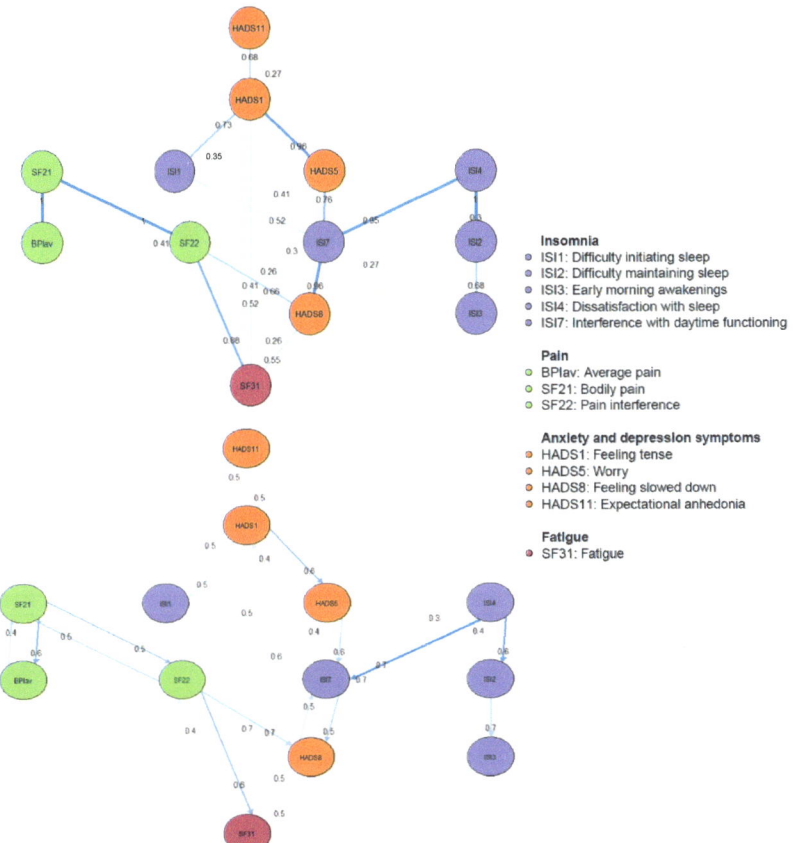

Figure 3. Bayesian networks, directed acyclic graphs: directional dependence relations. In the top panel, edge thickness signifies the magnitude of the Bayesian Information Criterion (BIC). Thicker edges indicate that the removal of the edge would significantly impact model fit. On the panel underneath, edge thickness represents the probability of the direction depicted.

4. Discussion

This exploratory study aimed to understand how symptoms of nCSP and insomnia are connected by examining the interconnections, strengths, and directions of symptoms of sleep, pain, fatigue, anxiety and depression. Another aim was to identify the key symptoms, shed light on the bidirectional nature of the nCSP-insomnia relationship, and elucidate whether one condition exacerbates the other.

Previous research showed that sleep quality reduces pain thresholds, and perpetuates pain symptoms and vice versa [2,8–12]. Thus, symptoms can be considered as constitutive components of a disorder, actively influencing and maintaining each other through direct causal interactions [19,20]. We found only one direct link between sleep and pain, namely, between average pain and difficulties maintaining sleep. This amount of connections between sleep and pain symptoms might be explained by important differences between how patients perceive various symptoms and objectively measured symptoms. For example, differences arise in the measurement of sleep when comparing self-reported data and PSG data [49]. Furthermore, the link between average pain and difficulties maintaining sleep was rather weak. The strength of the association is not fully in accordance to previous studies, suggesting a stronger association [8,11]. The strongest links were found between symptoms in the same cluster, which implicates that symptoms have a high probability of covarying because they form an active part of the disorder [20]. Other relatively strong edges emerged between "Feeling slowed down" and "Interference with daytime functioning". This is in line with the finding that people with insomnia might be more vulnerable to symptoms of anxiety and depression, because contrary to insomnia symptoms, improvement in these symptoms did not predict a change in pain symptoms [8,10,12].

Symptoms of anxiety and depression are suggested to partially mediate the relationship between pain and sleep [14]. In line with this, we found that the pain and sleep clusters were indirectly linked through the cluster of anxiety and depression, suggesting a mediating role. Symptoms of anxiety and depression are more strongly connected to the symptoms of sleep. Also, contrary to the symptoms of sleep, pain symptoms are not situated in the cascade of expectational anhedonia, tension, and worry in the DAGs. Thus, persons with nCSP and comorbid insomnia who score high on the ISI items are more likely to score high on the HADS items. In other words, insomnia symptoms might be the consequence of the variables of the anxiety and depression cluster in the sleep and pain network, while pain symptoms might not be. In addition, all symptoms of anxiety and depression are rather parent nodes instead of the consequence of another node. The only exception is feeling slowed down, which is suggested to be a terminal node in the DAGs with direct connections from both insomnia and pain symptoms (i.e., pain interference and interference with daytime interference due to insomnia). In other words, feeling slowed down might be the consequence of interference in functioning due to both pain and sleep. Here, pain interference might be a greater contributor to feeling slowed down in comparison to interference due to insomnia. This is in line with previous research that suggests that improvements in depression symptoms do not predict change in pain, as the presence of feeling slowed down implies the presence of pain interference more strongly than vice versa [8,10,12]. Besides feeling slowed down, fatigue also appeared as a terminal node, as the presence of fatigue more likely implies the presence of pain interference instead of interference in daytime functioning due to insomnia. This is in agreement with fatigue being a prevalent complaint of both insomnia and chronic pain patients, and with the patient-determined success criterion for the treatment of nCSP being the reduction of fatigue [13,16]. Another possible explanation might be an increase in Type II errors due to the very small sample size in the present study and/or the limited measure of fatigue, in which there is no distinction between mental and physical fatigue [24,41].

Additionally, a network analysis allowed us to reveal the key symptoms in the network. First, the most central constructs in the pain–sleep network were pain interference, bodily pain, interference in daytime functioning, and tension. These constructs were not significantly more central compared to each other in this network. This might be explained by the effect of a small sample size on the accuracy of centrality measures [24]. Nevertheless, when a construct is connected to many nodes but only explains a little of the variance in the network, this construct might not be as important to the network as a construct which is connected to only two other constructs but explains half of the variance in the network [21]. In this network, the most central constructs, except for tension, were most determined by all other constructs in the network, which suggests some importance to the network, which is, however, limited due to the lack of a large sample size. Furthermore, it is important to note that the networks do not include all possible variables. Missing nodes include stressors other than pain, predisposing factors for insomnia (e.g., arousal predisposition), fear of pain, etc. These and other "etiological nodes" are unobserved and thus latent in this network structure [20]. Although they probably influence other variables, they do not form an unobserved variable that influences all other variables. Thus, they do not qualify to portray latent variables as implied in the latent variable model [20].

Previous research showed a reciprocal relation between sleep disturbance and chronic pain, where sleep quality reduces pain thresholds, and perpetuates pain symptoms and vice versa [2,8–12]. Nonetheless, sleep disturbance is considered a better predictor of pain than vice versa. This is suggested to lie in the contribution of insomnia in the abnormalities in pain processing and hyper analgesic responses [8,9]. Contrary to the cited research, we found only one direct, but weak, link between sleep and pain, in which pain is more strongly connected to sleep compared to the other way around. This means that the difficulties maintaining sleep might be a consequence of the presence of average pain in nCSP patients with comorbid insomnia [21]. In other words, if difficulties maintaining sleep are present, it more strongly implies the presence of average pain than vice versa. One potential explanation for the lack of strong, direct associations between sleep and pain might be that anxiety, depression, and fatigue mediate the link between insomnia and nCSP [10,12,13]. Another possible explanation is that questionnaires assess the subjective experience of symptoms, which is different from the objective measurements of these symptoms, and might be subject to reporting biases [50,51].

Moreover, the symptoms of anxiety and depression are parent nodes instead of the consequence of another node. Only feeling slowed down might be the consequence of interference in functioning due to both pain and sleep. This aligns with the vulnerability model of tonic/phasic dopamine dysregulation, suggesting that irregularities in the mesolimbic dopamine system trigger insomnia, chronic pain, and depression symptoms [18]. Exacerbations of these symptoms create a feedback loop, which further contributes to dopamine dysregulation [14].

4.1. Strengths and Limitations

This study has several strengths. Firstly, to our knowledge, no research using network analysis on an item level and directed acyclic graphs has been applied to assess comorbidity between nCSP and insomnia. This could potentially inspire further studies to examine the interrelations within a larger sample size, which is a crucial step in confirming the robustness and generalizability of our initial findings. Moreover, we used standardized questionnaires. Nevertheless, some limitations of our study can be mentioned. First, in terms of network analyses, our sample size is limited. This may have led to poor or acceptable (but not ideal) stability [24]. Therefore, the interpretation of this explorative study should be performed with care. Second, cross-sectional DAGs can only disclose directional dependence relations, but cannot confirm temporal precedence [22]. Third, the assumption of causal sufficiency and causal faithfulness in DAGs were violated in this study. In other words, not all common causes are integrated in the network [48]. This means that the estimated causal effects may be biased [48]. Adhering to these assumptions is challenging in psychological data, as it is difficult to retain information in questionnaires on the directionality of influence between symptoms and if there are latent variables underlying these symptoms [48]. Therefore, these assumptions, with the causal faithfulness in particular, are likely to be violated [48].

Implications

These directional dependence relations among symptoms should not be mistaken for causal relations either. Consequently, straightforward implications for treatment in individuals with nonspecific chronic spinal pain and comorbid insomnia are difficult to obtain. Early research on network analysis suggested that symptoms high on strength centrality could be potential therapeutic targets for intervention [52,53]. Later work on network analysis urged to reconsider this, as drawing this conclusion comes with caveats [54]. Therefore, our presented results are best understood as a step toward theories about the structure of the causal system underlying nonspecific chronic spinal pain and comorbid insomnia [22]. In other words, these results could be seen as simplified, preliminary depictions of potential causal associations, which, in turn, could lead to clearer, straightforward implications for diagnosis, assessment, and treatment [22].

5. Conclusions

The current study explored the interrelationships between pain and sleep in nonspecific chronic spinal pain patients with comorbid insomnia, identifying key symptoms and highlighting the role of anxiety, depression, and fatigue. Contrary to previous research, no direct, or at best weak, links were found between sleep and pain, except average pain and difficulties maintaining sleep. Anxiety and depression were more strongly connected to sleep compared to pain, suggesting their influence in the sleep–pain relationship. Furthermore, feeling slowed down and fatigue emerged as terminal nodes, also implying their role as consequences of the network. Overall, we contributed insights into the interrelationship between sleep and pain. Future studies could further explore the interrelations in nonspecific chronic spinal pain patients.

Supplementary Materials: The following supporting information can be downloaded at: https://www.mdpi.com/article/10.3390/jcm13051452/s1, Table S1: Edge-weights matrix: regularized GGM; Figure S1: Edge-weights stability graph: GGM; Figure S2: Centrality stability graph: GGM; Figure S3: Edge-weights difference test: GGM; Figure S4: Spearman correlation network; Figure S5: Centrality difference test: GGM.

Author Contributions: Conceptualization, Z.G. and O.M.; Data curation, T.B. and E.V.L.; Formal analysis, Z.G.; Investigation, T.B.; Methodology, Z.G.; Resources, M.M. (Mira Meeus), L.D., K.I., B.C., M.M. (Maarten Moens), J.N. and O.M.; Supervision, L.D.B. and O.M.; Visualization, Z.G.; Writing—original draft, Z.G.; Writing—review and editing, T.B., E.V.L., A.M., M.M. (Mira Meeus), L.D., K.I., B.C., A.R., M.M. (Maarten Moens), J.N., L.D.B. and O.M. All authors have read and agreed to the published version of the manuscript.

Funding: This research was funded by the Research Foundation Flanders (Fonds voor Wetenschappelijk Onderzoek Vlaanderen), Belgium (FWO-TBM project no. T001117N). The funder played no role in the design, conduct, or reporting of this study. Thomas Bilterys his research is supported by the EUTOPIA Science and Innovation Fellowship Programme and funded by the European Union Horizon 2020 programme under the Marie Sklodowska-Curie granr agreement No 945380. This article reflects only the author's view and the Research Executive Agency is not responsible for any use that may be made of the information it contains. It was furthermore supported by the Strategic Research Program SRP90 ('Pain Never Sleeps: Unravelling the Sleep–Pain Interaction in Patients with Chronic Pain') funded by the research council of the Vrije Universiteit Brussel, Brussels, Belgium.

Institutional Review Board Statement: Not applicable.

Informed Consent Statement: Not applicable.

Data Availability Statement: No new data were created or analyzed in this study. Data sharing is not applicable to this article.

Conflicts of Interest: The authors declare no conflicts of interest.

References

1. Bilterys, T.; Siffain, C.; De Maeyer, I.; Van Looveren, E.; Mairesse, O.; Nijs, J.; Meeus, M.; Ickmans, K.; Cagnie, B.; Goubert, D.; et al. Associates of Insomnia in People with Chronic Spinal Pain: A Systematic Review and Meta-Analysis. *J. Clin. Med.* **2021**, *10*, 3175. [CrossRef]
2. Kelly, G.A.; Blake, C.; Power, C.K.; O'keeffe, D.; Fullen, B.M. The Association Between Chronic Low Back Pain and Sleep A Systematic Review. *Clin. J. Pain* **2011**, *27*, 169–181. [CrossRef] [PubMed]
3. Malfliet, A.; Bilterys, T.; Van Looveren, E.; Meeus, M.; Danneels, L.; Ickmans, K.; Cagnie, B.; Mairesse, O.; Neu, D.; Moens, M. et al. The added value of cognitive behavioral therapy for insomnia to current best evidence physical therapy for chronic spinal pain: Protocol of a randomized controlled clinical trial. *Braz. J. Phys. Ther.* **2019**, *23*, 62–70. [CrossRef]
4. Langevin, H.M.; Sherman, K.J. Pathophysiological model for chronic low back pain integrating connective tissue and nervous system mechanisms. *Med. Hypotheses* **2007**, *68*, 74–80. [CrossRef]
5. Dekker, K.; Blanken, T.F.; Van Someren, E.J.W. Insomnia and personality—A network approach. *Brain Sci.* **2017**, *7*, 28. [CrossRef]
6. Hu, F.; Li, L.; Huang, X.; Yan, X.; Huang, P. Symptom distribution regularity of insomnia: Network and spectral clustering analysis. *JMIR Med. Inform.* **2020**, *8*, e16749. [CrossRef] [PubMed]
7. Jansson-Fröjmark, M.; Boersma, K. Bidirectionality between pain and insomnia symptoms: A prospective study. *Br. J. Health Psychol.* **2012**, *17*, 420–431. [CrossRef]
8. Agmon, M.; Armon, G. Increased Insomnia Symptoms Predict the Onset of Back Pain among Employed Adults. *PLoS ONE* **2014**, *9*, e103591. [CrossRef] [PubMed]
9. Haack, M.; Simpson, N.; Sethna, N.; Kaur, S.; Mullington, J. Sleep deficiency and chronic pain: Potential underlying mechanisms and clinical implications. *Neuropsychopharmacology* **2020**, *45*, 205–216. [CrossRef]

10. Koffel, E.; Kroenke, K.; Bair, M.J.; Leverty, D.; Polusny, M.A.; Krebs, E.E. The bidirectional relationship between sleep complaints and pain: Analysis of data from a randomized trial. *Health Psychol.* **2016**, *35*, 41–49. [CrossRef]
11. Skarpsno, E.S.; Mork, P.J.; Marcuzzi, A.; Lund Nilsen, T.I.; Meisingset, I. Subtypes of insomnia and the risk of chronic spinal pain: The HUNT study. *Sleep Med.* **2021**, *85*, 15–20. [CrossRef]
12. Herrero Babiloni, A.; de Koninck, B.P.; Beetz, G.; de Beaumont, L.; Martel, M.O.; Lavigne, G.J. Sleep and pain: Recent insights, mechanisms, and future directions in the investigation of this relationship. *J. Neural Transm.* **2020**, *127*, 647–660. [CrossRef]
13. de la Vega, R.; Racine, M.; Castarlenas, E.; Solé, E.; Roy, R.; Jensen, M.P.; Miró, J.; Cane, D. The Role of Sleep Quality and Fatigue on the Benefits of an Interdisciplinary Treatment for Adults With Chronic Pain. *Pain Pract.* **2019**, *19*, 354–362. [CrossRef] [PubMed]
14. Dzierzewski, J.M.; Ravyts, S.; Griffin, S.C.; Rybarczyk, B. Sleep and Pain: The Role of Depression. *Curr. Sleep Med. Rep.* **2019**, *5*, 173–180. [CrossRef]
15. De Baets, L.; Runge, N.; Labie, C.; Mairesse, O.; Malfliet, A.; Verschueren, S.; Van Assche, D.; de Vlam, K.; Luyten, F.P.; Coppieters, I.; et al. The interplay between symptoms of insomnia and pain in people with osteoarthritis: A narrative review of the current evidence. *Sleep Med. Rev.* **2023**, *70*, 101793. [CrossRef] [PubMed]
16. Brown, J.L.; Edwards, P.S.; Atchison, J.W.; Lafayette-Lucey, A.; Wittmer, V.T.; Robinson, M.E. Defining patient-centered, multidimensional success criteria for treatment of chronic spine pain. *Pain Med.* **2008**, *9*, 851–862. [CrossRef] [PubMed]
17. Miller, C.B.; Gu, J.; Henry, A.L.; Davis, M.L.; Espie, C.A.; Stott, R.; Heinz, A.J.; Bentley, K.H.; Goodwin, G.M.; Gorman, B.S.; et al. Feasibility and efficacy of a digital CBT intervention for symptoms of Generalized Anxiety Disorder: A randomized multiple-baseline study. *J. Behav. Ther. Exp. Psychiatry* **2021**, *70*, 101609. [CrossRef] [PubMed]
18. Mason, E.C.; Harvey, A.G. Insomnia before and after treatment for anxiety and depression. *J. Affect. Disord.* **2014**, *168*, 415–421. [CrossRef]
19. Fried, E.I.; Cramer, A.O.J. Illness pathways between eating disorder and post-traumatic stress disorder symptoms: Understanding comorbidity with network analysis. *Eur. Eat. Disord. Rev.* **2019**, *27*, 147–160.
20. Cramer, A.O.J.; Waldorp, L.J.; Van Der Maas, H.L.J.; Borsboom, D. Comorbidity: A network perspective. *Behav. Brain Sci.* **2010**, *33*, 137–150. [CrossRef]
21. Robinaugh, D.J.; Millner, A.J.; McNally, R.J. Identifying highly influential nodes in the complicated grief network. *J. Abnorm. Psychol.* **2016**, *125*, 747–757. [CrossRef]
22. McNally, R.J.; Robinaugh, D.J.; Deckersbach, T.; Sylvia, L.G.; Nierenberg, A.A. Estimating the Symptom Structure of Bipolar Disorder via Network Analysis: Energy Dysregulation as a Central Symptom. *J. Psychopathol. Clin. Sci.* **2022**, *131*, 86–97. [CrossRef] [PubMed]
23. Borsboom, D.; Cramer, A.O.J. Network analysis: An integrative approach to the structure of psychopathology. *Annu. Rev. Clin. Psychol.* **2013**, *9*, 91–121. [CrossRef] [PubMed]
24. Epskamp, S.; Borsboom, D.; Fried, E.I. Estimating psychological networks and their accuracy: A tutorial paper. *Behav Res Methods* **2018**, *50*, 195–212. [CrossRef] [PubMed]
25. Epskamp, S.; Waldorp, L.J.; Mõttus, R.; Borsboom, D. The Gaussian Graphical Model in Cross-Sectional and Time-Series Data. *Multivar. Behav. Res.* **2018**, *53*, 453–480. [CrossRef]
26. Epskamp, S.; Maris, G.K.J.; Waldorp, L.J.; Borsboom, D. Network Psychometrics. *arXiv* **2016**, arXiv:1609.02818. [CrossRef]
27. Dalege, J.; Borsboom, D.; van Harreveld, F.; van der Maas, H.L.J. Network Analysis on Attitudes: A Brief Tutorial. *Soc. Psychol. Personal. Sci.* **2017**, *8*, 528–537. [CrossRef] [PubMed]
28. Iber, C. The AASM manual for the scoring of sleep and associated events: Rules, terminology, and technical specification. (No Title). 2007. Available online: https://scholar.google.com/citations?view_op=view_citation&hl=en&user=mLTec7cAAAAJ&citation_for_view=mLTec7cAAAAJ:tOudhMTPpwUC (accessed on 15 January 2024).
29. Jun, J.; Park, C.G.; Kapella, M.C. Psychometric properties of the Insomnia Severity Index for people with chronic obstructive pulmonary disease. *Sleep Med.* **2022**, *95*, 120–125. [CrossRef]
30. Hinz, A.; Glaesmer, H.; Brähler, E.; Löffler, M.; Engel, C.; Enzenbach, C.; Hegerl, U.; Sander, C. Sleep quality in the general population: Psychometric properties of the Pittsburgh Sleep Quality Index, derived from a German community sample of 9284 people. *Sleep Med.* **2017**, *30*, 57–63. [CrossRef]
31. Morin, C.M.; Drake, C.L.; Harvey, A.G.; Krystal, A.D.; Manber, R.; Riemann, D. Insomnia disorder. *Nat. Rev. Dis. Primers* **2015**, *1*, 15026.
32. Sateia, M.J. International classification of sleep disorders. *Chest* **2014**, *146*, 1387–1394. [CrossRef]
33. Riemann, D.; Espie, C.A.; Altena, E.; Arnardottir, E.S.; Baglioni, C.; Bassetti, C.L.A.; Bastien, C.; Berzina, N.; Bjorvatn, B.; Dikeos, D.; et al. The European Insomnia Guideline: An update on the diagnosis and treatment of insomnia. *J. Sleep Res.* **2023**, *32*, e14035.
34. Mairesse, O.; Damen, V.; Newell, J.; Kornreich, C.; Verbanck, P.; Neu, D. The Brugmann Fatigue Scale: An Analogue to the Epworth Sleepiness Scale to Measure Behavioral Rest Propensity. *Behav. Sleep Med.* **2019**, *17*, 437–458. [CrossRef]
35. Johns, M.W. A New Method for Measuring Daytime Sleepiness: The Epworth Sleepiness Scale. *Sleep* **1991**, *14*, 540–545. [CrossRef]
36. Morin, C.M.; Vallières, A.; Ivers, H. Dysfunctional Beliefs and Attitudes about Sleep (DBAS): Validation of a Brief Version (DBAS-16). *Sleep* **2007**, *30*, 1547–1554. [CrossRef] [PubMed]
37. Atkinson, T.M.; Rosenfeld, B.D.; Sit, L.; Mendoza, T.R.; Fruscione, M.; Lavene, D.; Shaw, M.; Li, Y.; Hay, J.; Cleeland, C.S.; et al. Using confirmatory factor analysis to evaluate construct validity of the Brief Pain Inventory (BPI). *J. Pain Symptom Manag.* **2011**, *41*, 558–565. [CrossRef] [PubMed]

38. Kregel, J.; Vuijk, P.J.; Descheemaeker, F.; Keizer, D.; Van Der Noord, R.; Nijs, J.; Cagnie, B.; Meeus, M.; van Wilgen, P. The Dutch Central Sensitization Inventory (CSI). *Clin. J. Pain* **2016**, *32*, 624–630. [CrossRef]
39. Ware, J.E.; Sherbourne, C.D. The MOS 36-Item Short-Form Health Survey (SF-36): I. Conceptual Framework and Item Selection. *Med. Care* **1992**, *30*, 473–483. [CrossRef] [PubMed]
40. Stern, A.F. The Hospital Anxiety and Depression Scale. *Occup. Med.* **2014**, *64*, 393–394. [CrossRef]
41. Hevey, D. Network analysis: A brief overview and tutorial. *Health Psychol. Behav. Med.* **2018**, *6*, 301–328. [CrossRef]
42. Levinson, C.A.; Brosof, L.C.; Vanzhula, I.; Christian, C.; Jones, P.; Rodebaugh, T.L.; Langer, J.K.; White, E.K.; Warren, C.; Weeks, J.W.; et al. Social anxiety and eating disorder comorbidity and underlying vulnerabilities: Using network analysis to conceptualize comorbidity. *Int. J. Eat. Disord.* **2018**, *51*, 693–709. [CrossRef]
43. Heeren, A.; Mouguiama-Daouda, C.; McNally, R.J. A network approach to climate change anxiety and its key related features. *J. Anxiety Disord.* **2023**, *93*, 102625. [CrossRef] [PubMed]
44. Tsang, S.; Royse, C.F.; Terkawi, A.S. Guidelines for developing, translating, and validating a questionnaire in perioperative and pain medicine. *Saudi J. Anaesth.* **2017**, *11*, S80–S89. [CrossRef]
45. Borsboom, D.; Deserno, M.K.; Rhemtulla, M.; Epskamp, S.; Fried, E.I.; McNally, R.J.; Robinaugh, D.J.; Perugini, M.; Dalege, J.; Costantini, G.; et al. Network analysis of multivariate data in psychological science. *Nat. Rev. Methods Primers* **2021**, *1*, 58. [CrossRef]
46. Carter, J.S.; Rossell, D.; Smith, J.Q. Partial Correlation Graphical LASSO. *arXiv* **2021**, arXiv:arXiv:2104.10099. [CrossRef]
47. Heeren, A.; Bernstein, E.E.; McNally, R.J. Bridging maladaptive social self-beliefs and social anxiety: A network perspective. *J. Anxiety Disord.* **2020**, *74*, 102267. [CrossRef] [PubMed]
48. Briganti, G.; Scutari, M.; Mcnally, R.J. A tutorial on Bayesian Networks for psychopathology researchers. Network theory comes with. *Psychol. Methods* **2022**, *28*, 947–961. [CrossRef]
49. Lehrer, H.M.; Yao, Z.; Krafty, R.T.; Evans, M.A.; Buysse, D.J.; Kravitz, H.M.; Matthews, K.A.; Gold, E.B.; Harlow, S.D.; Samuelsson, L.B.; et al. Comparing polysomnography, actigraphy, and sleep diary in the home environment: The Study of Women's Health Across the Nation (SWAN) Sleep Study. *Sleep Adv.* **2022**, *3*, zpac001. [CrossRef] [PubMed]
50. Alsaadi, S.M.; McAuley, J.H.; Hush, J.M.; Lo, S.; Bartlett, D.J.; Grunstein, R.R.; Maher, C.G. The bidirectional relationship between pain intensity and sleep disturbance/quality in patients with low back pain. *Clin. J. Pain* **2014**, *30*, 755–765. [CrossRef]
51. Tang, N.K.Y.; Goodchild, C.E.; Sanborn, A.N.; Howard, J.; Salkovskis, P.M. Deciphering the temporal link between pain and sleep in a heterogeneous chronic pain patient sample: A multilevel daily process study. *Sleep* **2012**, *35*, 675–687. [CrossRef]
52. McNally, R.J.; Robinaugh, D.J.; Wu, G.W.Y.; Wang, L.; Deserno, M.K.; Borsboom, D. Mental disorders as causal systems: A network approach to posttraumatic stress disorder. *Clin. Psychol. Sci.* **2015**, *3*, 836–849. [CrossRef]
53. Briganti, G.; Kornreich, C.; Linkowski, P. A network structure of manic symptoms. *Brain Behav.* **2021**, *11*, e02010. [CrossRef] [PubMed]
54. Rodebaugh, T.L.; Tonge, N.A.; Piccirill, M.L.; Fried, E.; Horenstein, A.; Morrison, A.S.; Goldin, P.G.; James, J.L.; Michelle, H. Fernandez, K.C.; et al. Does centrality in a cross-sectional network suggest intervention targets for social anxiety disorder? *J. Consult. Clin. Psychol.* **2018**, *86*, 831–844. [CrossRef] [PubMed]

Disclaimer/Publisher's Note: The statements, opinions and data contained in all publications are solely those of the individual author(s) and contributor(s) and not of MDPI and/or the editor(s). MDPI and/or the editor(s) disclaim responsibility for any injury to people or property resulting from any ideas, methods, instructions or products referred to in the content.

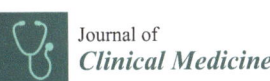

Article

Are Sleep Aids Associated with the Severity of Attention Deficit Hyperactivity Disorder Symptoms in Adults Screened for Insomnia? A Cross-Sectional Study

Omar Gammoh [1,*], Abdelrahim Alqudah [2], Esam Qnais [3], Alaa A. A. Aljabali [4], Ammena Y. Binsaleh [5] and Sireen Abdul Rahim Shilbayeh [5]

[1] Department of Clinical Pharmacy and Pharmacy Practice, Faculty of Pharmacy, Yarmouk University, Irbid 21163, Jordan
[2] Department of Clinical Pharmacy and Pharmacy Practice, Faculty of Pharmaceutical Sciences, The Hashemite University, Zarqa 13133, Jordan; abdelrahim@hu.edu.jo
[3] Department of Biology and Biotechnology, Faculty of Science, The Hashemite University, Zarqa 13133, Jordan; esamqn@hu.edu.jo
[4] Department of Pharmaceutics and Pharmaceutical Technology, Faculty of Pharmacy, Yarmouk University, Irbid 21163, Jordan; alaaj@yu.edu.jo
[5] Department of Pharmacy Practice, College of Pharmacy, Princess Nourah Bint Abdulrahman University, P.O. Box 84428, Riyadh 11671, Saudi Arabia; aysaleh@pnu.edu.sa (A.Y.B.); ssabdulrahim@pnu.edu.sa (S.A.R.S.)
* Correspondence: omar.gammoh@yu.edu.jo

Abstract: (1) **Background**: Attention Deficit Hyperactivity Disorder (ADHD)-like symptoms and insomnia are closely related. The present study examined whether the use of different sleep aids was related to severe ADHD-like symptoms in Jordanian adults screened for insomnia. (2) **Methods**: This cross-sectional study used predefined inclusion criteria. The severity of ADHD was assessed using the validated Arabic version of the Adult ADHD Self-Report Scale. (3) **Results**: Data were analyzed from 244 subjects who met the inclusion criteria for severe insomnia, of which 147 (65.3%) reported not using any sleep aid, 50 (22.3%) reported using homeopathy remedies as sleep aids, and 41 (18.3%) reported using over-the-counter antihistamines as sleep aids. Regression analysis revealed that the use of such sleep aids—namely, "homeopathy herbal remedies" and "over-the-counter antihistamines"—was not associated ($p > 0.05$) with ADHD-like symptoms. However, "age above 31 years old" was significantly associated ($B = -3.95$, $t = -2.32$, $p = 0.002$) with lower ADHD severity, while the "diagnosis with chronic diseases" was significantly associated ($B = 4.15$, $t = 1.99$, $p = 0.04$) with higher ADHD severity. (4) **Conclusions**: Sleep aids are not associated with ADHD-like symptoms in adults. More research is required to uncover the risk factors for adult ADHD, especially insomnia.

Keywords: Attention Deficit Hyperactivity Disorder (ADHD); insomnia; sleep aids; Adult ADHD Self-Report Scale

1. Introduction

Attention Deficit Hyperactivity Disorder (ADHD), a complex neurodevelopmental condition, has been a focal point for researchers and clinicians for the past 30 years. This novel research draws upon extensive expertise to explore recent scientific findings on ADHD, highlighting the intricate interplay of genetic, environmental, and neurological factors in its manifestation. Globally, adult ADHD prevalence ranges from 2.5% to 4.4%, with the National Institute of Mental Health (NIMH) reporting an overall prevalence of 4.4%, with higher rates in males (5.4%) than females (3.2%) [1]. A 2021 global meta-analysis reported a prevalence of 2.58% for persistent adult ADHD and 6.76% for symptomatic adult ADHD [2]. Also, adult ADHD is a significant burden in different countries; for example, adult ADHD prevails in 5.2% of the population in the United States, 6% in Northern Ireland, 1.8% in China, and 2.9% in Canada [3,4].

Adult ADHD can exert a notable influence on diverse facets of an individual's life, including their career trajectory, interpersonal relationships, and various other aspects of daily life [5].

Insomnia is prevalent among adults with ADHD [6]. The relationship between ADHD and sleep problems is reciprocal, with ADHD symptoms potentially causing insomnia and improved sleep quality possibly alleviating ADHD symptoms. Factors such as side effects of ADHD medications, hyperactivity, and restlessness may contribute to sleep disturbances in individuals with ADHD [7]. Research suggests that bright light therapy in the morning has promise in improving sleep-related issues in adults with ADHD. Those dealing with both ADHD and insomnia must maintain good sleep hygiene, consider behavioral therapies, and consult a doctor for appropriate treatment options when needed.

Insomnia, an integral part of the mental health spectrum, is highly affected by stressful environmental events or the distressing, violent, and aggressive content of war, which has a global impact on mental health [8,9]. It has been reported that there is a link between the severity of ADHD symptoms, different dimensions of ADHD symptoms, symptoms of insomnia, and sleep duration in adults. This underscores the recurring connection between noteworthy ADHD symptoms, specifically inattention and hyperactivity, and insomnia symptoms, alongside changes in sleep duration. There is an urgent need to evaluate and address insomnia and changes in sleep duration among adults with ADHD [10]. Other studies have reported sleep-related factors in adults diagnosed with ADHD. They revealed that approximately 85% of participants experienced excessive daytime sleepiness or subpar sleep quality, with prevalent issues including difficulty falling asleep initially, disrupted sleep, and feeling excessively warm during sleep. Moreover, distinctions emerged between individuals who predominantly exhibited inattentive symptoms (ADHD-I) and those with combined symptoms (ADHD-C). The ADHD-I group reported lower sleep quality and increased fatigue compared to the ADHD-C group, with a notable interplay between subtype and gender influencing perceptions of fatigue [11].

The potential link between the use of sleep aids, specifically antihistamines, and the risk of ADHD in children is an evolving research topic. The impact of such aids on adult ADHD has not been adequately studied [12]. It is recognized that the relationship between sleep and ADHD is complex. Children with ADHD experiencing persistent sleep-onset insomnia may find melatonin beneficial in improving both the time taken to initiate sleep and overall duration of sleep. Sleep problems are common in adults with ADHD, and the interplay between ADHD and sleep disturbances is bidirectional [7]. While the precise effects of sleep aids on adult ADHD are not fully understood, it is crucial to consider potential consequences, including those of antihistamines, and seek guidance from healthcare professionals when addressing sleep issues in the context of ADHD [13].

The relationship between adult ADHD and sleep aid use has yet to be explored in Jordan. Nevertheless, existing research has investigated the impact of stimulant medications on the sleep patterns of adults with ADHD [7,12]. These investigations suggest that stimulant medications may induce side effects that lead to insomnia and compromise the overall quality of sleep in this population. Therefore, it is crucial for clinicians to monitor and address the potential impact of stimulant medications on sleep dynamics in adults with ADHD.

The principal objective of this study is to examine the potential correlation between self-administration of sleep aids and various clinical factors leading to heightened ADHD symptoms in a cohort of individuals in Jordan who underwent screening for insomnia during the ongoing war in Gaza. This study aims to address a significant void in the current academic literature by specifically focusing on the interconnection between self-medication practices involving sleep aids, coupled with other clinical variables, and the emergence of elevated ADHD symptoms. Existing studies have primarily explored ADHD symptoms and their associations with sleep-related challenges, as shown in the SWOT analysis in Table 1. However, there is a noteworthy deficiency in the research conducted in the Jordanian context, particularly concerning self-medication practices with sleep aids. Through this inquiry, we aim to provide innovative perspectives that not only enhance the prevailing comprehension of ADHD symptoms in the context of insomnia, but also furnish healthcare practitioners, policymakers, and researchers engaged with the Jordanian population with valuable insights. The study is meticulously crafted to bridge this gap and deliver a more comprehensive understanding of the complex relationship between self-medication practices, clinical factors, and ADHD symptoms, thereby contributing to the intellectual discourse in this specialized domain. The study's characteristics are evaluated in Table 1 below.

Table 1. Evaluation of study characteristics—strengths, weaknesses, opportunities, and threats in investigating the relationship between sleep aids and ADHD in the Jordanian population.

Strengths	Weaknesses	Opportunities	Threats
- Addresses a specific gap in the literature by focusing on the Jordanian population, providing a unique and context-specific perspective on the relationship between sleep aids and ADHD.	- Limited Generalizability: Focus on the Jordanian population may restrict applicability to other cultural or demographic contexts.	- Informing Interventions: Positive findings could contribute to targeted interventions for Jordanian individuals experiencing ADHD symptoms in the context of insomnia.	- External Factors: Economic, political, or social factors in Jordan may impact study implementation and outcomes.
- Comprehensive approach: Aims to explore the multifaceted relationship by considering various clinical factors, contributing to a more thorough understanding of the subject.	- Potential Bias: Self-reporting of sleep aid use and ADHD symptoms may introduce bias as participants may not accurately recall or report their behaviors.	- Guidance for Healthcare Practices: Study can guide healthcare practitioners in addressing self-medication practices with sleep aids and managing ADHD symptoms.	- Limited Participation: Difficulty in recruiting a representative sample may compromise study validity and applicability.
- Practical Implications: Findings could have practical applications for healthcare practitioners, policymakers, and researchers, offering valuable insights for potential interventions or guidelines.	- Complexity of Variables: Involvement of various clinical factors may introduce complexity, making it challenging to isolate the direct impact of sleep aids on ADHD symptoms.	- Foundation for Further Research: Successful completion could lay the groundwork for further research exploring similar relationships in diverse populations or refining methodologies.	- Ethical Considerations: Ensuring participant confidentiality and addressing potential ethical concerns related to self-medication practices and mental health disclosures is crucial.

2. Materials and Methods
2.1. Study Design and Recruitment

This cross-sectional study recruited a cohort of Jordanians using a convenient sampling method. The web-based study was approved by Yarmouk University IRB committee (protocol code 692) on 28 December 2023. All the participants read about and agreed to be enrolled in the study by choosing the option "I agree to participate" on the informed consent form provided by the corresponding author. All of the data obtained were anonymous. The study instrument was uploaded onto a Google Form, and the link was distributed on various social media platforms in Jordan. Data were collected during January 2024. The sample size was based on a confidence level of 95%, a confidence interval of 5%, and an estimated population size of 10 million. This resulted in the need to recruit 384 participants before the inclusion criteria could be applied.

2.2. Inclusion Crieria

Exclusive consideration was given to adults who reported clinically significant insomnia, as determined by the Arabic version of the Insomnia Severity Index (ISI-A) [14]. Developed by Morin et al. [15], the ISI-A consists of seven questions with Likert-type responses and produces a score in the range of 0 to 28. A cut-off score exceeding 14 is established as an indicative threshold for severe insomnia symptoms.

2.3. Study Instrument
Covariates

Demographic data and relevant information were systematically recorded, encompassing variables such as gender (male or female), age (below 30 years old or 30 years old and above), marital status (single or married), number of family members (fewer than five members or five members or more), the highest level of education completed (bachelor's degree or graduate studies), smoking status (smoker or non-smoker), participants' affiliation with the medical field (affiliated or unaffiliated), employment status (employed or unemployed), and any previous diagnoses of chronic conditions, with a primary focus on hypertension, diabetes, and dyslipidemia. To determine the specific self-medication practices related to sleep aids within the study sample, participants were given the autonomy to choose one or more options from the following categories: "homeopathy herbal remedies", "over-the-counter sedating antihistamines", or "never used any sleep aid".

2.4. Outcome Variable
ADHD Symptom Severity

The assessment of symptoms resembling ADHD was carried out using the validated Arabic version of the Adult ADHD Self-Report Scale-V1.1 (ASRS), which comprises an 18-item scale. Aligned with the diagnostic criteria outlined in the Diagnostic and Statistical Manual of Mental Disorders (DSM) for ADHD, this scale produces a score in the range of 0 to 72, with higher scores indicating more severe symptoms [16,17].

2.5. Data Analysis

Frequencies and percentages were used to describe the demographics of the study sample. To determine which covariates are associated with ADHD severity, a preliminary univariate linear regression analysis was carried out, and potential confounders showing $p < 0.1$ were included in the multivariate linear regression analysis. Confidence intervals were set at 95%, and significance was set at $p < 0.05$. Data were analyzed using SPSS version 21.

3. Results

3.1. Response Rate

A total of 542 participants were approached, 487 agreed to participate, and 263 participants did not meet the inclusion criteria for insomnia; therefore, the data from 224 participants were analyzed.

3.2. Study Sample Demographics

The demographic analysis of the study resulted in insightful findings about the participant profile. Out of the initial 542 participants approached, 487 consented to participate, resulting in a comprehensive dataset of 224 participants after excluding 263 individuals who did not meet the inclusion criteria for insomnia. Among the participants, 156 (69.6%) were females, highlighting a significant gender disparity in favor of women. It is worth noting that 156 (69.6%) participants were single, indicating a substantial proportion of unmarried individuals in the study. From a demographic standpoint, 118 (52.7%) participants reported having five or more family members, a factor that warrants consideration due to its potential implications for sleep patterns and overall well-being. Additionally, the employment status of the participants was significant, with 155 (69.2%) reporting unemployment, which may have an impact on lifestyle and sleep routines. Regarding lifestyle factors, 90 (40.2%) participants disclosed being smokers, providing further insight into potential contributors to sleep patterns and overall health. Shifting the focus to the usage of sleep aids, 147 (65.3%) participants reported not using any sleep aids, indicating a prevalent reliance on natural sleep patterns. Among those who did use sleep aids, 50 (22.3%) opted for homeopathic remedies, revealing a preference for natural or alternative approaches to sleep management. Moreover, 41 (18.3%) participants reported using over-the-counter antihistamines as sleep aids, highlighting a segment of the population that relies on pharmaceutical options. These meticulous demographic details and sleep aid usage patterns present a nuanced portrayal of the study population, establishing a solid foundation for a comprehensive analysis of the correlation between sleep aid utilization and ADHD-like symptoms in adults grappling with insomnia. The detailed results are succinctly summarized in Table 2.

Table 2. Sample characteristics ($n = 224$).

Factor	Category	n (%)
Sex	Male	68 (30.4)
	Female	156 (69.6)
Age	Below 30 years	148 (66.1)
	31 years and above	76 (33.9)
Marital status	Single	156 (69.6)
	Married	68 (30.4)
Family members	Fewer than 5	106 (47.3)
	5 or more	118 (52.7)
Highest education	Bachelor's	190 (84.8)
	Graduate studies	34 (15.2)
Employment status	Unemployed	155 (69.2)
	Employed	69 (30.8)
Are you studying?	no	131 (58.5)
	yes	93 (41.5)
Are you in the medical field?	No	106 (47.3)
	Yes	118 (52.7)
Smoking status	Non-smoker	134 (59.8)
	Smoker	90 (40.2)
Diagnosed with chronic diseases?	No	183 (81.7)
	Yes	41 (18.3)
I use herbal homeopathy preparations for sleep		50 (22.3)
I use over-the-counter antihistamines for sleep (sedating antihistamines)		41 (18.3)
I do not use any sleep aids		147 (65.3)

3.3. Correlates of ADHD Symptom Severity

The severity of ADHD symptoms was evaluated using the validated Arabic version of the ASRS. Higher scores indicated greater ADHD severity. To identify factors associated with ADHD, an initial univariate linear regression analysis was conducted (as shown in Table 3), followed by a comprehensive multivariate analysis with ADHD as the dependent variable (Table 4). It is worth noting that the final model was adjusted for both "age" and "diagnosis with chronic diseases". The results of the analysis revealed a significant association between individuals aged above 31 years and lower ADHD severity (B = −3.95, t = −2.32, p = 0.002). Conversely, a diagnosis of chronic diseases was significantly associated with higher ADHD severity (B = 4.15, t = 1.99, p = 0.04), suggesting a notable correlation between health conditions and the manifestation of ADHD-like symptoms. Interestingly, the utilization of sleep aids did not demonstrate any statistically significant association with ADHD-like symptoms. Therefore, it can be inferred that the presence or absence of sleep aid usage did not impact the severity of ADHD symptoms in the study population. These findings, systematically presented in Tables 3 and 4, contribute to a comprehensive understanding of the factors influencing ADHD severity in the cohort under study. They have implications for both clinical considerations and future research endeavors.

Table 3. Univariate linear regression for ADHD symptoms as the dependent variable.

Factor	B	t	p	95% CI
Female gender	2.67	1.51	0.13	−0.80–6.13
Age above 31 years	−3.53	−2.08	0.03 *	−6.88−−0.19
Married	−3.89	−2.29	0.02 *	−7.33−−0.45
Five or more family members	1.54	0.95	0.34	−1.66–4.74
Graduate studies	−2.64	−1.17	0.24	−7.09–1.80
Employed	0.47	0.26	0.79	3.0–3.93
Student	1.00	0.61	0.54	−2.24–4.26
Medical field	2.67	1.65	0.10	−0.51–5.86
Smoking	2.99	1.81	0.07	−0.25–6.23
Diagnosed with chronic diseases	3.55	1.70	0.09	−0.56–7.67
I use herbal homeopathy preparations for sleep	−1.32	−0.68	0.49	−5.16–2.51
I use over-the-counter antihistamines for sleep	1.37	0.65	0.51	−2.76–5.51
I do not use any sleep aids	−0.53	−0.31	0.75	−3.91–2.83

The ADHD symptom severity was assessed using the validated Arabic version of ASRS. B: beta, t: t-value, CI: confidence interval, * p < 0.05.

Table 4. Multivariate linear regression for ADHD symptom severity as the dependent variable.

Factor	B	t	p	95% CI
Age above 31 years	−3.95	−2.32	0.002	−7.31−−0.60
Diagnosis with a chronic disease	4.15	1.99	0.04	0.05–8.26

The ADHD symptom severity was assessed using the validated Arabic version of ASRS. CI: confidence interval.

4. Discussion

The objective of this investigation was to examine the potential association between the use of sleep aids, such as antihistamines or homeopathic remedies, and ADHD-like symptoms in adults being screened for insomnia. Our findings indicate that the sleep aids used by the participants did not have any significant correlation with the severity of ADHD symptoms. However, we did find other factors that were strongly correlated with the severity of ADHD symptoms in the study population. Younger age was significantly associated with more severe ADHD symptoms, highlighting the importance of age in understanding the manifestation of ADHD-like symptoms. Additionally, individuals with chronic illnesses were also linked to higher ADHD symptom severity, suggesting a potential interaction between health conditions and the severity of ADHD symptoms in adults with insomnia. These findings provide valuable insights into the complex relationship between sleep aid usage, demographic factors, and the severity of ADHD-like symptoms. Further research is needed to fully explore the connections among these variables and gain a more comprehensive understanding of the factors influencing ADHD symptomatology in individuals undergoing insomnia screening.

The use of antihistamines is well established for dermatological and respiratory allergies. Previous studies have related the use of antihistamines to an increased risk of ADHD symptoms in children. For example, in one pilot retrospective study on children aged 6–12 years with atopic dermatitis, the study concluded that previous exposure to antihistamines was associated with about a two-fold incidence of developing ADHD symptoms [18]. In addition, another recent cohort study recruiting data from >40,000 children has demonstrated that children exposed to antihistamines have a 35% risk of ADHD [19]. Our findings revealed that antihistamines were not associated with ADHD symptom severity. Although the precise explanation of this finding requires additional larger-scale studies, several factors can provide insights. One possible explanation is that the metabolism and the distribution of these sedating antihistamines are different in adults, thus leading to alteration in the drug's bioavailability and therefore its concentration in the site of action, in this case, the central nervous system. Another explanation is that the present study examines the whole class of antihistamines without stratification of each medication in this group. Perhaps future studies could study the effect of individual antihistamines such as chlorpheniramine or diphenhydramine that are frequently consumed as over-the-counter sleep aids [20]. Another explanation is that other demographics and clinical factors such as the chronic diseases of the participants and the chronically received medications could interfere with cognition. This is one of few studies that brings adult ADHD under the spotlight. Previous studies have indicated that the vast majority of adults with ADHD are underdiagnosed and undertreated [2]. The proper diagnosis of ADHD is quite challenging as it overlaps with other psychiatric illnesses, such as depression and anxiety [21], especially in developing countries such as Jordan where these disorders are stigmatized.

In the present study, it was found that participants aged above 30 years old were less likely to experience symptoms of severe ADHD and vice versa, i.e., participants with an age lower than 30 years were at a lower risk of developing severe ADHD symptoms. This supports previous research showing that a majority of adults with ADHD had symptoms in their youth [22]. The higher prevalence of ADHD symptoms in younger adults may be due to the challenges they face in educational settings, which are more demanding compared to the flexible working environments available to adults [23,24]. These findings emphasize the importance of considering developmental stages and environmental factors when studying ADHD symptoms in adults. Further research is needed to explore the relationship between age, environmental stressors, and ADHD symptoms for a more comprehensive understanding of this complex interaction.

The presence of chronic diseases in our cohort was predictive of higher ADHD symptom severity. In the present study, chronic diseases were mainly cardiovascular (hypertension and diabetes). This finding is consistent with previous studies. For example, a large cross-sectional study confirmed a positive association between cardiovascular disease and ADHD [25]. In addition, a recent study revealed that 46% of patients with type 2 diabetes reported ADHD-like symptoms [26]. This could be explained by the fact that subjects with ADHD-like symptoms could adopt negative behaviors that exacerbate metabolic control [27]. Moreover, both cardiovascular and cognitive impairment could share common ground in stress and inflammation [28,29]. Additionally, the medications used for chronic diseases could predispose patients to cognitive and mood disturbances [30,31]. The cross-talk between cardiovascular diseases and ADHD symptoms has common ground in biological backgrounds. This includes implication of the immune system, inflammatory cascades, neuromodulation, and hormonal dysregulation mainly in the hypothalamic–pituitary–adrenal (HPA) axis, as in [32]. In addition, the daily consumption of cardiovascular medications could predispose people to cognitive-related symptoms, although research in this area did not result in conclusive results [30,33]. This represents an attractive and challenging topic to investigate due to the complexity of the demographical, clinical, and patient's intrinsic factors. For example, some studies could not relate the use of cardiovascular medications to impaired cognition [33]; on the other hand, another investigation that recruited a cohort of geriatric subjects concluded that the use of cardiovascular medications was significantly associated with lower incidence of cognitive impairment [34].

This study contributes to the limited literature focusing on adult ADHD symptoms. Although the idea, the validated scales, and the statistical model are all considered strengths, the study has some limitations. The symptoms of ADHD were not assessed by a professional psychiatrist. Although the study used a validated scale, as in previous studies, the self-reported scales could be associated with high prevalence rates compared to accurate medical or psychiatric diagnosis. Another limitation is that the study findings cannot be generalized to the Jordanian population as this would require an expansion of the study sample. In addition, the study did not examine other potential confounders, such as lifestyle, food and water consumption, the potential effect of chronic medication, and others. Also, the design did not include the names of specific antihistamines or herbal remedies. Furthermore, the cross-sectional design did not allow for the examination of the causal relationship between sleep aids and ADHD symptoms.

5. Conclusions

Our study investigated the correlation between the use of sleep aids and ADHD-like symptoms in adults with insomnia in Jordan. Among the 244 participants who had severe insomnia, 65.3% did not use any sleep aids. Homeopathic remedies were chosen by 22.3% of participants, while 18.3% used over-the-counter antihistamines. Contrary to our initial hypothesis, regression analysis did not find any statistically significant relationship between the use of sleep aids (specifically homeopathic herbal remedies and over-the-counter antihistamines) and ADHD-like symptoms ($p > 0.05$). However, certain demographic factors did affect the severity of ADHD symptoms. Participants being over the age of 31 showed a significant association with lower ADHD severity, while a diagnosis of chronic diseases was linked to higher ADHD severity. The analysis of demographic data provided intriguing insights into the study population. The higher prevalence of females and unmarried individuals suggests that gender and marital status may influence the severity of ADHD. Furthermore, information on family size, employment status, and smoking habits helped us gain a better understanding of the cohort. Correlational analysis, including univariate and multivariate linear regression, further supported the impact of age and chronic diseases on ADHD severity. These findings underscore the importance of considering both demographic and health-related factors when evaluating adult ADHD. Importantly, the use of sleep aids did not contribute to ADHD-like symptoms in this particular population. These results contribute to the existing research on adult ADHD and emphasize the significance of age and health status in determining the severity of symptoms. Future studies should explore the intricate relationship between insomnia, sleep aids, and ADHD in diverse populations to gain further insights into potential risk factors and approaches to treatment.

Author Contributions: Conceptualization, O.G., A.A. and S.A.R.S.; methodology, A.A.A.A.; software, A.Y.B.; validation, O.G., A.A. and A.Y.B.; formal analysis, E.Q.; investigation, A.A.A.A.; resources, O.G.; data curation, E.Q.; writing—original draft preparation, O.G. and A.Y.B.; writing—review and editing, A.A., O.G. and S.A.R.S.; visualization, A.A.A.A. and S.A.R.S.; supervision, E.Q.; project administration, O.G.; funding acquisition, A.Y.B. and S.A.R.S. All authors have read and agreed to the published version of the manuscript.

Funding: Princess Nourah bint Abdulrahman University Researchers Supporting Project Number (PNURSP2024R419).

Institutional Review Board Statement: The study was conducted in accordance with the Declaration of Helsinki and approved by the Institutional Review Board of Yarmouk University (protocol code 692 on 28 December 2023).

Informed Consent Statement: Informed consent was obtained from all subjects involved in the study.

Data Availability Statement: Data associated with this publication will be available from the corresponding author upon request.

Acknowledgments: The current work was supported by Princess Nourah bint Abdulrahman University Researchers Supporting Project Number (PNURSP2024R419), Princess Nourah bint Abdulrahman University, Riyadh, Saudi Arabia. The corresponding author would like to thank Nour, Yasmina, Suza, and Sama for their support.

Conflicts of Interest: The authors declare no conflicts of interest.

References

1. Forbes, F. Attention deficit hyperactivity disorder (ADHD). *J.-R. Coll. Physicians Edinb.* **2006**, *36*, 315.
2. Song, P.; Zha, M.; Yang, Q.; Zhang, Y.; Li, X.; Rudan, I. The prevalence of adult attention-deficit hyperactivity disorder: A global systematic review and meta-analysis. *J. Glob. Health* **2021**, *11*, 04009. [CrossRef] [PubMed]
3. Fayyad, J.; Sampson, N.A.; Hwang, I.; Adamowski, T.; Aguilar-Gaxiola, S.; Al-Hamzawi, A.; Andrade, L.H.S.G.; Borges, G.; de Girolamo, G.; Florescu, S.; et al. The descriptive epidemiology of DSM-IV Adult ADHD in the World Health Organization World Mental Health Surveys. *ADHD Atten. Deficit Hyperact. Disord.* **2017**, *9*, 47–65. [CrossRef] [PubMed]
4. Hesson, J.; Fowler, K. Prevalence and correlates of self-reported ADD/ADHD in a large national sample of Canadian adults. *J. Atten. Disord.* **2018**, *22*, 191–200. [CrossRef] [PubMed]
5. Ginapp, C.M.; Greenberg, N.R.; Macdonald-Gagnon, G.; Angarita, G.A.; Bold, K.W.; Potenza, M.N. The experiences of adults with ADHD in interpersonal relationships and online communities: A qualitative study. *SSM-Qual. Res. Health* **2023**, *3*, 100223. [CrossRef]
6. Fadeuilhe, C.; Daigre, C.; Richarte, V.; Grau-López, L.; Palma-Álvarez, R.F.; Corrales, M.; Ramos-Quiroga, J.A. Insomnia disorder in adult attention-deficit/hyperactivity disorder patients: Clinical, comorbidity, and treatment correlates. *Front. Psychiatry* **2021**, *12*, 663889. [CrossRef]
7. Surman, C.B.H.; Walsh, D.M. Managing sleep in adults with ADHD: From science to pragmatic approaches. *Brain Sci.* **2021**, *11*, 1361. [CrossRef]
8. Andén-Papadopoulos, K. Body horror on the internet: US soldiers recording the war in Iraq and Afghanistan. *Media Cult. Soc.* **2009**, *31*, 921–938. [CrossRef]
9. Bresheeth, H. Projecting trauma. *Third Text* **2006**, *20*, 57–71. [CrossRef]
10. Wynchank, D.; Ten Have, M.; Bijlenga, D.; Penninx, B.W.; Beekman, A.T.; Lamers, F.; de Graaf, R.; Kooij, J.J.S. The association between insomnia and sleep duration in adults with attention-deficit hyperactivity disorder: Results from a general population study. *J. Clin. Sleep Med.* **2018**, *14*, 349–357. [CrossRef] [PubMed]
11. Yoon, S.Y.R.; Jain, U.R.; Shapiro, C.M. Sleep and daytime function in adults with attention-deficit/hyperactivity disorder: Subtype differences. *Sleep Med.* **2013**, *14*, 648–655. [CrossRef]
12. Stein, M.A.; Weiss, M.; Hlavaty, L. ADHD treatments, sleep, and sleep problems: Complex associations. *Neurotherapeutics* **2012**, *9*, 509–517. [CrossRef]
13. Hvolby, A. Associations of sleep disturbance with ADHD: Implications for treatment. *ADHD Atten. Deficit Hyperact. Disord.* **2015**, *7*, 1–18. [CrossRef]
14. Suleiman, K.H.; Yates, B.C. Translating the insomnia severity index into Arabic. *J. Nurs. Scholarsh.* **2011**, *43*, 49–53. [CrossRef]
15. Morin, C. Insomnia: Psychological Assessment and Management. 1993. Available online: https://psycnet.apa.org/record/1993-98362-000 (accessed on 2 November 2019).
16. El Hayek, G.; Saab, D.; Farhat, C.; Krayem, Z.; Karam, E. Adult ADHD in the Arab world: A review. *Arch. Psychol.* **2019**, *3*, 1–23. [CrossRef]
17. Alharbi, N.; Alotaibi, K.F.; Althaqel, G.K.; Alasmari, N.Y.; Alahmari, A.F.; Alasmari, O.Y.; Alshahrani, M.S.; Alghamdi, L.A.; Alrashed, H.A.; Shugair, N.A. Adult Attention Deficit Hyperactivity Disorder (ADHD) among residents of Saudi Arabia: A cross-sectional study. *Eur. Rev. Med. Pharmacol. Sci.* **2023**, *27*, 10935–10943. [PubMed]
18. Schmitt, J.; Buske-Kirschbaum, A.; Tesch, F.; Trikojat, K.; Stephan, V.; Abraham, S.; Bauer, A.; Nemat, K.; Plessow, F.; Roessner, V. Increased attention-deficit/hyperactivity symptoms in atopic dermatitis are associated with history of antihistamine use. *Allergy* **2018**, *73*, 615–626. [CrossRef] [PubMed]
19. Fuhrmann, S.; Tesch, F.; Romanos, M.; Abraham, S.; Schmitt, J. ADHD in school-age children is related to infant exposure to systemic H1-antihistamines. *Allergy* **2020**, *75*, 2956–2957. [CrossRef]
20. Gammoh, O.S.; Al-Smadi, A.; Turjman, C.; Mukattash, T.; Kdour, M. Valerian: An underestimated anxiolytic in the community pharmacy? *J. Herb. Med.* **2016**, *6*, 193–197. [CrossRef]
21. Torgersen, T.; Gjervan, B.; Rasmussen, K. ADHD in adults: A study of clinical characteristics, impairment and comorbidity. *Nord. J. Psychiatry* **2006**, *60*, 38–43. [CrossRef] [PubMed]
22. Hutt Vater, C.; DiSalvo, M.; Ehrlich, A.; Parker, H.; O'Connor, H.; Faraone, S.V.; Biederman, J. ADHD in Adults: Does Age at Diagnosis Matter? *J. Atten. Disord.* **2024**, *28*, 10870547231218450. [CrossRef]

23. Lasky, A.K.; Weisner, T.S.; Jensen, P.S.; Hinshaw, S.P.; Hechtman, L.; Arnold, L.E.; Murray, D.W.; Swanson, J.M. ADHD in context: Young adults' reports of the impact of occupational environment on the manifestation of ADHD. *Soc. Sci. Med.* **2016**, *161*, 160–168. [CrossRef]
24. Whalen, C.K. ADHD treatment in the 21st century: Pushing the envelope. *J. Clin. Child Adolesc. Psychol.* **2001**, *30*, 136–140. [CrossRef]
25. Xu, G.; Snetselaar, L.G.; Strathearn, L.; Ryckman, K.; Nothwehr, F.; Torner, J. Association between history of attention-deficit/hyperactivity disorder diagnosis and cardiovascular disease in US adults. *Health Psychol.* **2022**, *41*, 693. [CrossRef] [PubMed]
26. Dehnavi, A.Z.; Zhang-James, Y.; Draytsel, D.; Carguello, B.; Faraone, S.V.; Weinstock, R.S. Association of ADHD symptoms with type 2 diabetes and cardiovascular comorbidities in adults receiving outpatient diabetes care. *J. Clin. Transl. Endocrinol.* **2023**, *32*, 100318. [CrossRef] [PubMed]
27. Nylander, C.; Lindström, K.; Khalifa, N.; Fernell, E. Previously undiagnosed attention-deficit/hyperactivity disorder associated with poor metabolic control in adolescents with type 1 diabetes. *Pediatr. Diabetes* **2018**, *19*, 816–822. [CrossRef] [PubMed]
28. Uzun, N.; Akıncı, M.A.; Alp, H. Cardiovascular disease risk in children and adolescents with attention deficit/hyperactivity disorder. *Clin. Psychopharmacol. Neurosci.* **2023**, *21*, 77. [CrossRef] [PubMed]
29. Saccaro, L.F.; Schilliger, Z.; Perroud, N.; Piguet, C. Inflammation, anxiety, and stress in attention-deficit/hyperactivity disorder. *Biomedicines* **2021**, *9*, 1313. [CrossRef] [PubMed]
30. Gammoh, O.; Bjørk, M.-H.; Al Rob, O.A.; AlQudah, A.R.; Hani, A.B.; Al-Smadi, A. The association between antihypertensive medications and mental health outcomes among Syrian war refugees with stress and hypertension. *J. Psychosom. Res.* **2023**, *168*, 111200. [CrossRef] [PubMed]
31. Gammoh, O.; Al-Smadi, A.; Mansour, M.; Ennab, W.; AL Hababbeh, S.; Al-Taani, G.; Alsous, M.; Aljabali, A.A.A.; Tambuwala, M.M. The relationship between psychiatric symptoms and the use of levetiracetam in people with epilepsy. *Int. J. Psychiatry Med.* **2023**, 00912174231206056. [CrossRef]
32. Li, L.; Yao, H.; Zhang, L.; Garcia-Argibay, M.; Du Rietz, E.; Brikell, I.; Solmi, M.; Cortese, S.; Ramos-Quiroga, J.A.; Ribasés, M. et al. Attention-deficit/hyperactivity disorder is associated with increased risk of cardiovascular diseases: A systematic review and meta-analysis. *JCPP Adv.* **2023**, *3*, e12158. [CrossRef] [PubMed]
33. Rohde, D.; Hickey, A.; Williams, D.; Bennett, K. Cognitive impairment and cardiovascular medication use: Results from wave 1 of The Irish Longitudinal Study on Ageing. *Cardiovasc. Ther.* **2017**, *35*, e12300. [CrossRef] [PubMed]
34. Liu, E.; Dyer, S.M.; O'Donnell, L.K.; Milte, R.; Bradley, C.; Harrison, S.L.; Gnanamanickam, E.; Whitehead, C.; Crotty, M. Association of cardiovascular system medications with cognitive function and dementia in older adults living in nursing homes in Australia. *J. Geriatr. Cardiol. JGC* **2017**, *14*, 407. [PubMed]

Disclaimer/Publisher's Note: The statements, opinions and data contained in all publications are solely those of the individual author(s) and contributor(s) and not of MDPI and/or the editor(s). MDPI and/or the editor(s) disclaim responsibility for any injury to people or property resulting from any ideas, methods, instructions or products referred to in the content.

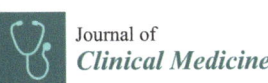

Review

Insomnia in Forensic Detainees: Is Salience Network the Common Pathway for Sleep, Neuropsychiatric, and Neurodegenerative Disorders?

Adonis Sfera [1,2,*], Kyle A. Thomas [1], Isaac A. Ogunjale [1], Nyla Jafri [1] and Peter G. Bota [2]

- [1] Department of Psychiatry, Patton State Hospital, University of California, Riverside, CA 92521, USA
- [2] School of Medicine, California University of Science and Medicine, Colton, CA 92324, USA
- * Correspondence: adois.sfera@dsh.ca.gov

Highlights:

What are the main findings?

- SN dysfunction is the common denominator of insomnia, schizophrenia (SCZ), and frontotemporal dementia behavioral variant (bvFTD).

What is the implication of the main finding?

- The diagnosis of bvFTD is often missed or misdiagnosed in forensic institutions.
- To ensure adequate placement and treatment planning, courts and clinicians require education to differentiate bvFTD from SCZ.

Abstract: Forensic hospitals throughout the country house individuals with severe mental illness and history of criminal violations. Insomnia affects 67.4% of hospitalized patients with chronic neuropsychiatric disorders, indicating that these conditions may hijack human somnogenic pathways. Conversely, somnolence is a common adverse effect of many antipsychotic drugs, further highlighting a common etiopathogenesis. Since the brain salience network is likely the common denominator for insomnia, neuropsychiatric and neurodegenerative disorders, here, we focus on the pathology of this neuronal assembly and its likely driver, the dysfunctional neuronal and mitochondrial membrane. We also discuss potential treatment strategies ranging from membrane lipid replacement to mitochondrial transplantation. The aims of this review are threefold: 1. Examining the causes of insomnia in forensic detainees with severe mental illness, as well as its role in predisposing them to neurodegenerative disorders. 2. Educating State hospital and prison clinicians on frontotemporal dementia behavioral variant, a condition increasingly diagnosed in older first offenders which is often missed due to the absence of memory impairment. 3. Introducing clinicians to natural compounds that are potentially beneficial for insomnia and severe mental illness.

Keywords: Von Economo neuron; interoceptive awareness; frontotemporal dementia behavioral variant; phenazines

1. Introduction

One of the most common sleep disorders in the United States, primary insomnia, is usually defined as long sleep latency, difficulty staying asleep, prolonged nighttime wakefulness, and/or early morning awakening [1]. In prison, approximately 60% of inmates experience insomnia, a prevalence 6–10 times higher than in the population at large [2]. Moreover, insomnia is present in 67.4% of hospitalized patients with severe mental illness, suggesting that the pathways of sleep and neuropathology are highly intertwined [3].

Forensic psychiatric hospitals admit patients with schizophrenia (SCZ) or schizophrenia-like disorders (SLDs) and criminal violations. Insomnia is common in this population and failure to address this condition may increase healthcare expenditure due to medical complications, including metabolic, cardiovascular, and neurodegenerative disorders.

The salience network (SN), comprised of the anterior insular cortex (AIC), anterior cingulate cortex (ACC) and several subcortical nodes, has recently been implicated in the etiopathogenesis of insomnia, SCZ, and neurodegenerative disorders [4–9]. SN is comprised of Von Economo neurons (VENs), a special class of large, spindle-shaped cells found only in humans and superior mammals that are believed to drive empathy, social awareness, and emotional intelligence [10].

At the molecular level, incarceration, insomnia, and severe mental illness have been associated with premature cellular senescence, a phenotype marked by increased intracellular iron and mitochondrial damage [11–18]. Premature cellular senescence is driven by the aryl hydrocarbon receptor (AhR), expressed in neuronal cytosol and mitochondria [19–21]. Senescent cells upregulate intracellular iron which, in the proximity of cytosolic fats, increases the risk of lipid peroxidation and neuronal demise by ferroptosis [22–24]. Ferroptosis is a programmed cell death induced by iron in the context of antioxidant failure marked by the depletion of glutathione peroxidase-4 (GPX-4) [25,26]. GPX-4 is a mitochondrial enzyme which averts ferroptosis by repairing the oxidized phospholipids and cholesterol in mitochondrial and neuronal membranes [27]. Ferroptosis causes mitochondrial swelling, loss of cristae, dissipation of the membrane potential, as well as an increase in membrane permeability, changes that ultimately lead to mitochondrial loss [28]. Mitochondrial dysfunction and loss drive cellular senescence, a phenotype found in insomnia, severe mental illness and frontotemporal lobar degeneration (FTLD) [29–32]. In addition, insomnia, SCZ, and frontotemporal dementia (FTD) have been connected to impaired phagocytosis of senescent cells by natural killer cells (NKCs) [33–35]. Accumulation of senescent cells due to accelerated aging and impaired removal leads to inflammation, a pathology encountered in sleep deprivation, severe mental illness and FTD [36–38]. Since mitochondria is a key driver of inflammation, dysfunction or loss of these organelles likely account for these pathologies [39,40].

To compensate for dysfunctional mitochondria, neurons import these organelles from glial cells, especially the astrocyte [41,42]. In large cells, such as VENs, mitochondria are more vulnerable to damage and autophagic elimination as they undergo more wear and tear during their journey through the long axons of these neurons [42]. Due to their small number (around 193,000) and their large sizes, VENs are more susceptible to plasma membrane oxidative stress, which may trigger significant pathology even after a limited neuronal loss, a pathology encountered in frontotemporal dementia behavioral variant (bvFTD) [43].

Since mitochondria are crucial for neuronal function, preserving the integrity of these organelles via membrane lipid replacement (MLR) and other natural strategies is of utmost importance. Microbial phenazines and the novel antioxidant phenothiazine derivatives offer new opportunities to combat insomnia, psychosis, and neurodegeneration at the level of cell and mitochondrial membranes.

1.1. Salienve Network in Sleep and Neuropathology

The SN is comprised of ACC and AIC which, along with subcortical nodes in the hypothalamus, thalamus, striatum, and midbrain, process salient stimuli [44,45]. SN functions as a switch between exteroception and interoception or central executive network (CEN) and default mode network (DMN), depending on stimulus relevance [46]. Switching from CEN to DMN and vice versa is impaired in severe mental illness, insomnia, and neurodegenerative disorders [47]. Several antipsychotic drugs are known to lower the salience assignment to objects and events, likely restoring SN function, which, in turn, may ameliorate insomnia and psychosis [48].

The SN harbors VENs, which are large, corkscrew neurons located in layer V of the AIC and ACC. These non-telencephalic cells are believed to drive prosocial cognition, empathy, and emotional intelligence. As parts of the SN, VENs respond to endogenous or exogenous stimuli in the order of priority. VENs are selectively eliminated in bvFTD, a disorder marked by criminal violations, lack of empathy, poor insight, and sleep impairment [49–53]. In forensic institutions, bvFTD is increasingly diagnosed in older first offenders with no previous criminal history and often coexists with insomnia and altered eating habits.

Under physiological circumstances, sleep is driven by the ventrolateral preoptic nucleus (VLPO) of the anterior hypothalamus which releases inhibitory neurotransmitters, including γ-aminobutyric acid (GABA), and galanin [54]. The opposing system, orexin (hypocretin) neurons in the lateral hypothalamus, inhibits VLPO [55–57]. In addition, orexin/hypocretin neurons induce wakefulness by blocking melanin concentrating hormone (MCH), a somnogen released by the hypothalamus and zona incerta [58,59]. Orexin and DA, the key players of saliency, have been implicated in the neuropsychiatric disorders associated with sleep disturbances, including narcolepsy, attention-deficit/hyperactivity disorder (ADHD), and Parkinson's disease (PD) [60]. Histamine is another wakefulness-promoting neurotransmitter implicated in SCZ and a novel target for treating negative and cognitive symptoms [61].

To better comprehend the pathogenesis of insomnia, it is necessary to study the pathways of wakefulness, a brain state driving self-awareness and probably consciousness [62]. Early studies on this subject have focused on the locus coeruleus, midbrain tegmentum, pons, and parabrachial nucleus, as neurons in these regions are active during wakefulness [63,64]. In the early 1900s, while studying encephalitis lethargica, Constantin von Economo found that lesions in the posterior hypothalamus were associated with sleep, hypothesizing that this area contained the "center of wakefulness" [65–67].

Fatal familial insomnia (FFI), a rare autosomal dominant disease, is marked by hypometabolism and neuronal loss in the thalamus and ACC, linking this condition to the SN [68–72]. The role of SN in sleep physiology and pathology is further highlighted by the anesthetics, especially propofol, which lower salience processing, inducing sleep [68–78]. Moreover, recent studies on sleep-deprived human volunteers and patients with primary insomnia demonstrated altered connectivity in AIC, further linking SN to sleep and wakefulness [79,80]. Furthermore, several preclinical studies are in line with the findings in humans, implicating the SN in slumber homeostasis [74,81].

Aside from insomnia and neuropsychiatric pathology, the SN connectivity is disrupted in neurodegenerative disorders, including Alzheimer's disease (AD), Parkinson's disease (PD), and bvFTD, suggesting that insomnia and neuropathology are highly intertwined [82–86]. Indeed, dysfunctional AIC and ACC connectivity may account for the criminal violations in patients with bvFTD, in which breaking the law may often be the initial dementia symptom [87,88].

1.2. Salience Network in Frontotemporal Dementia Behavioral Variant

The second most common neurodegenerative disorder after AD, bvFTD, is marked by inappropriate emotional responses and disinhibited behaviors, often leading to criminal violations, as this pathology targets VENs selectively [52,89]. In forensic institutions, individuals with first incarceration after the age of 55 may suffer from bvFTD, an entity difficult to diagnose as the memory may remain intact for longer periods of time. As a result, bvFTD is often missed or misdiagnosed as antisocial personality disorder (APD), SCZ, or even major depressive disorder [90].

Over the past two decades, the number of senior first offenders has grown in parallel with the prevalence of young-onset dementia (YOD, emergence of symptoms before age 65), a subgroup of neurodegenerative disorders, which may include bvFTD [91,92]. Indeed, recent studies have revealed that the prevalence of bvFTD has increased from 15/100,000 in 2013 to 119 per 100,000 in 2021, mirroring the growing number of forensic detainees with this diagnosis [92,93].

Compared to AD, in which 12% of patients exhibit criminal behavior, bvFTD is associated with a crime rate of 54%, suggesting an acquired psychopathy [94]. Frontotemporal lobar degeneration (FTLD), the pathology driving bvFTD, is associated with impulsivity and criminal violations due to the paucity of "honesty cells", VENs [95]. The latter is likely due to the autophagy of damaged organelles traveling through the long VENs axons. Indeed, lysosomal aggregates, hallmarks of hyperactive autophagy, were demonstrated in the VENs derived from patients with bvFTD and SCZ, suggesting excessive mitophagy [95–97]. Depletion of VENs has been associated with a lack of empathy, aggressive behavior, and criminal violations documented in bvFTD and severe mental illness [51,52]. For example, homicide or attempted homicide have been documented in bvFTD, indicating that criminal behavior and murder can sometimes be the earliest manifestation of this disorder [98,99]. Since VENs are only present in large mammals, including humans, great apes, macaques, cetaceans, and elephants, but not in rodents, these cells are difficult to study in vivo [10]. VENs are larger than pyramidal neurons and drive interoceptive awareness, which is the ability to detect and process internal cues such as heartbeat, respiration and the overall visceral state [100,101]. VENs are components of the SN, an attention-shifting large neuronal assembly that can activate or silence CEN to DMN [102,103].

Recent transcriptomic studies found that VENs express monoaminergic proteins, including vesicular monoamine transporter 2 (VMAT2) and adrenergic receptor α-1A (ADRA1A), suggesting involvement in autonomic functions, including the circadian rhythm [104–106]. Indeed, impaired monoaminergic signaling has been documented in insomnia, bvFTD, SCZ, and SLDs, implicating VENs in these pathologies [107–111].

1.3. Sleep and Glial Cells

Astrocytes, the most numerous brain cells, communicate with each other via calcium waves, attaining synchronization with neurons and supporting slow-wave sleep [112,113]. Moreover, astrocytes release molecules, including adenosine, lactate, glutamate, GABA, and interleukin-1 (IL-1), which may indirectly influence the status of neuronal cells, inducing sleep [114].

Astrocytes are central to the neurovascular unit (NVU) and bridge the gap between the neuron and brain microvessels, regulating the flow of interstitial fluid through the aquaporin 4 (AQP-4) receptors [115] (Figure 1). The volume of the brain interstitial fluid (ISF) fluctuates in a circadian manner as it flows through the glymphatic system, a mechanism for clearing misfolded proteins during sleep [116]. The glymphatic system can also carry extracellular vesicles containing mitochondria from astrocytes to neurons [117]. Astrocytes support the neurons by generating GPX-4 to avert neuronal death by ferroptosis. GPX-4 functions to repair oxidized lipids and oxysterols, including 7-ketocholesterol (7KCl), toxins that disrupt plasma and mitochondrial membranes, triggering neuronal death [118]. Ferroptosis has been associated with sleep deprivation, indicating that neurons likely import GPX-4 during sleep [119]. As mitochondria play a key role in sleep homeostasis, insomnia may be the result of plasma or mitochondrial membrane oxidation. Indeed, it has been suggested that sleep is necessary for abrogating neuronal oxidative stress [120].

Intracellular iron is stored in ferritin and released for intracellular needs via ferritinophagy (ferritin autophagy) in lysosomes. Several antipsychotic drugs, including haloperidol, accumulate in lysosomes disrupting ferritinophagy, which, in turn, lowers intracellular iron, averting ferroptosis [121,122] (Figure 2). This may highlight a DA-independent, antipsychotic action of haloperidol, suggesting that dopaminergic blockade is not the only psychosis-deterring mechanism of this drug. Indeed, ferroptosis of hippocampal neurons, documented in AD and severe mental illness, is the likely cause of cognitive impairment and negative symptoms in these conditions [123,124]. Prolonged insomnia has been demonstrated to damage the astrocyte which, in turn, may trigger neuronal demise [125]. Moreover, chronic sleep loss was demonstrated to activate both astrocytes and microglia, turning these cells into neurotoxic phenotypes capable of eliminating healthy neurons and synapses [126–128].

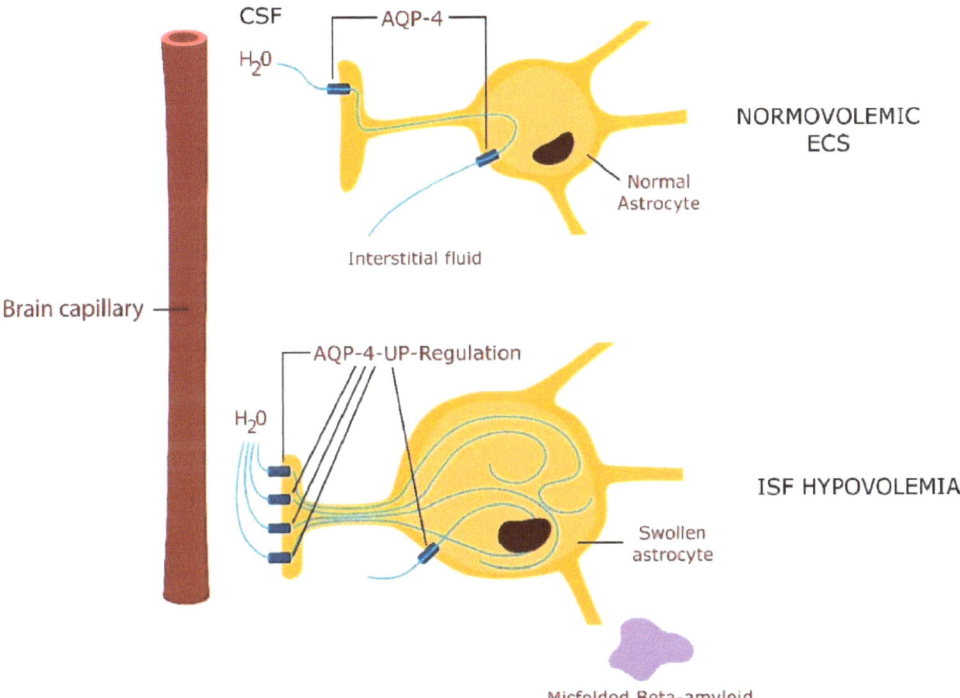

Figure 1. Astrocytes contact cerebral microvessels with their end-feet processes, delineating a pathway for the flow of extracellular fluid, known as the glymphatic system. The volume of interstitial fluid (ISF) in the brain parenchyma varies with the brain work. During high intensity work, AQP-4 water receptors are upregulated in the end-feet, pumping the ISF into astrocytes. This results in low ISF (hypovolemia). During sleep (low-intensity brain work), less ISF enters the astrocyte. The circulation of ISF clears the molecular debris (including beta amyloid) from the extracellular space.

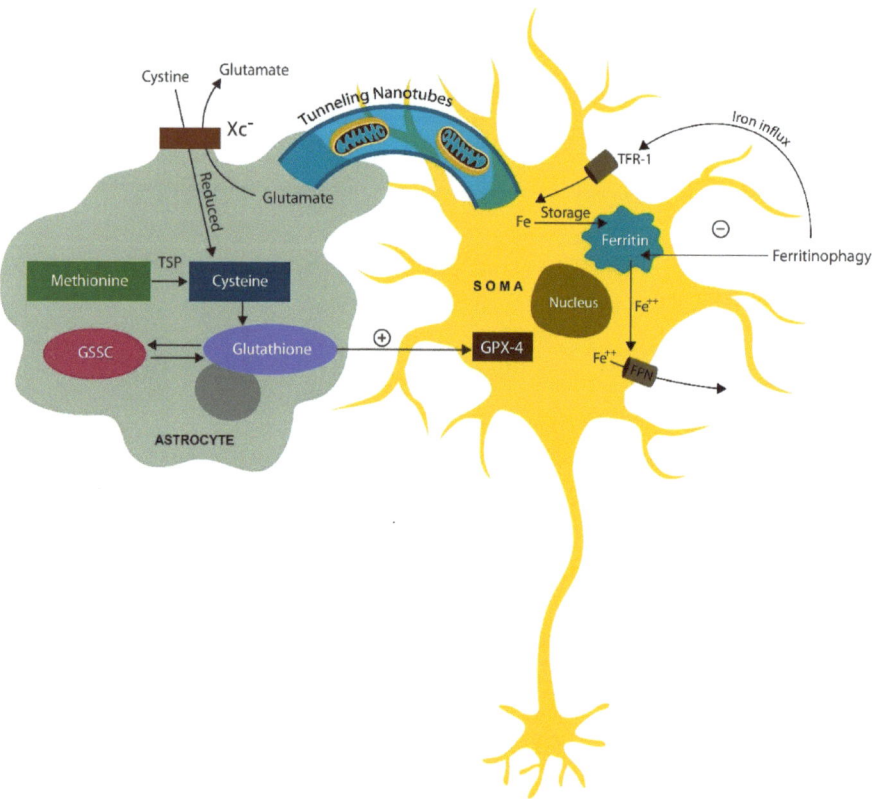

Figure 2. Astrocytes support the postmitotic, long-lived neurons by helping them avert death by ferroptosis and loss of mitochondria. The former is accomplished by exporting GPX-4 to neurons (to repair oxidized lipids), while the latter by exporting healthy mitochondria to neuronal cells (via tunneling nanotubules, extracellular vesicles, or cell–cell fusion). Astrocytes import cystine via cystine/glutamate antiporter (Xc-). Cystine is reduced to cysteine and generates glutathione and GPX-4 (which is transferred to neurons). Cysteine can also be derived from methionine, while glutathione can be generated from cysteine and glutathione disulfide (GSSC). In neurons, iron is stored in ferritin and, when needed, ferritin undergoes ferritinophagy (autophagy) in lysosomes, releasing free iron. Iron ingresses the neuron via transferrin receptor 1 (TRF-1), while the excess intracellular iron is eliminated via ferroportin.

2. Mitochondria and Aryl Hydrocarbon Receptor

Recent studies have implicated mitochondria in the pathophysiology of sleep and neurodegenerative disorders, while the role of these organelles in severe mental illness, including SCZ and SLDs, has been previously established [129,130]. AhR is the master regulator of cellular senescence, a phenotype conducive to aging and neurodegeneration and is expressed by the mitochondrion [19–21]. Oxidized lipids in the mitochondrial membrane are AhR ligands, which in conjunction with senescence-upregulated intracellular iron, can trigger ferroptosis and organelle demise [131–134]. Indeed, lipid peroxides and oxysterols, such as 7KCl, are mitoAhR ligands, contributing to mitochondrial dysfunction and autophagic elimination [135].

AhR is a xenobiotic sensor which regulates cytochrome p450 and binds the environmental toxin, dioxin (2,3,7,8-tetrachlorodibenzo-p-dioxin). Other AhR ligands include somnogens, such as phenazines, melatonin, and tryptophan derivatives, which participate in the physiology of sleep, wakefulness, and the circadian rhythm [136–138]. In addition, reactive oxygen species (ROS), known to induce sleep via a redox-sensitive potassium channel, are AhR ligands, bringing this transcription factor in the arena of slumber, mental illness, and neurodegeneration [131,139]. Indeed, microbial phenazines, including pyocyanin and 1-hydroxyphenazine, activate AhR, influencing the transcription of many genes, including those involved in sleep regulation [140,141].

The importance of mitochondria in sleep physiology is further substantiated by the organelle involvement in FFI, as well as in general anesthesia [142,143]. Indeed, general anesthetics are known to inhibit N-methyl-d-aspartate (NMDA) and α-amino-3-hydroxy-5-methyl-4-isoxazolepropionic acid (AMPA) glutamate receptors while stimulating GABA. NMDA and AMPA upregulate intracellular and mitochondrial calcium, inducing cell and organelle demise [144]. Interestingly, elevated mitochondrial calcium, a characteristic of prion diseases, may link these organelles to FFI [145,146]. Indeed, the prion peptide causes calcium inflow via L-type calcium channels, triggering neuronal damage and apoptosis [147]. In contrast, the typical antipsychotic, chlorpromazine, not only induces sleep, but also exerts anti-prion properties, probably by promoting autophagy of the misfolded protein [148–150].

Mitochondrial trafficking from astrocytes to neurons supports neuronal bioenergetic needs, especially in large pyramidal cells or VENs. Mitochondria can be imported via cell–cell fusion, tunneling nanotubes (cytoskeletal protrusions reaching to other cells), as well as transported by extracellular vesicles [151,152] (Figure 2). Moreover, astrocytes generate GPX-4 from cysteine obtained via the cystine/glutamate antiporter system (Xc−) or by transmethylation of methionine. Glutathione is generated from cysteine and glutathione disulfide (GSSC) [153] (Figure 2).

Mitochondrial trafficking as well as autophagy (mitophagy) occur during sleep, probably explaining the reason most living beings require rest [154]. Interestingly, serotonin (5-HT) promotes mitochondrial transport in hippocampal neurons, suggesting that antidepressant drugs, serotonin reuptake inhibitors (SSRIs), may "exert their action by supplying healthy mitochondria to stressed neurons [155]. This may imply that ROS accumulation during wakefulness may induce slumber to repair oxidized lipids and import mitochondria from glial cells [120,131,139]. In addition, the accumulation of intracellular microtubule-associated protein tau (MAPT) in VENs likely impairs mitochondrial transport, contributing to bvFTD pathogenesis [156].

2.1. Mitochondria-Protective Treatments

The key role of mitochondria in sleep disorders, SCZ, SLDs, and neurodegeneration, highlights the importance of mitoprotective approaches to resuscitate, replace, or increase the import of mitochondria from glial cells [157]. For example, treatment with SSRIs during the early stages of dementia may delay the onset of cognitive decline. Along this line, a recent study found that treatment with SSRIs slowed the conversion of mild cognitive impairment to frank dementia, suggesting that prophylactic treatment with these agents may be beneficial [158]. In addition, natural anti-ferroptosis drugs and iron chelators, such as halogenated phenazines, may improve the course of neurodegenerative disorders, suggesting novel therapeutic strategies [159,160].

2.2. Membrane Lipid Replacement (MLR)

MLR refers to the oral supplementation with natural cell membrane glycerophospholipids and kaempferol (3,4′,5,7-tetrahydroxyflavone), a natural flavonoid found in tea, broccoli, cabbage, kale, beans, endive, leek, tomato, strawberries, and grapes [161]. Kaempferol is a glycogen synthase kinase-3β (GSK-3β) inhibitor which prevents sleep deprivation-induced cognitive decline [162,163]. Like lithium and several antipsychotic drugs, kaempferol blocks GSK-3β, an enzyme previously implicated in SCZ and circadian rhythm disorders, suggesting that this natural compound may exert antipsychotic properties without the adverse effects of conventional therapeutics [164–167].

The aim of MLR + kaempferol is the gradual replacement of damaged phospholipids and oxysterols from neuronal and/or mitochondrial membranes with natural glycerophospholipids and a polyphenol. Indeed, oxidized membrane lipids have been implicated in SCZ, SLDs, insomnia, and neurodegeneration, while MLR and kaempferol offer a dual mechanism of action: (1) elimination of lipid peroxides and (2) GSK-3β inhibition [168]. Replacing oxidized plasma and/or mitochondrial membrane fats with healthy natural lipids averts deformation of the neuronal membrane and misalignment of neuroreceptors. Conversely, oxidized membrane lipids and ferroptosis alter the biophysical properties of membranes, disrupting neuronal functions [169].

2.3. Phenazines and Phenothiazine Derivatives

Several natural phenazines and phenothiazines are neuroprotective, improve sleep, and delay neurodegenerative processes. For example, geranyl-phenazine is a naural acetylcholinesterase inhibitor which exerts antipsychotic effects via muscarinic receptors. Indeed, a new class of antipsychotic drugs is currently being developed for SCZ and a patent exists for treating sleep disorders by upregulating acetylcholine [170–172] (WO2005016327A2). Other natural phenazines with neuroprotective functions include baraphenazines A–G fused compounds derived from Streptomyces sp. PU-10A which likely possess antipsychotic properties [173]. Moreover, several natural phenazines, including baraphenazines, leucanicidin and endophenasides, exert antimicrobial, anticancer activity, and very likely possess antipsychotic properties [173–175].

Natural antipsychotic and phytotherapeutic compounds are not only devoid of extrapyramidal adverse effects but more accepted by many patients who often dread or distrust pharmaceuticals.

Synthetic phenazine derivatives consist of over 6000 compounds, exerting antimicrobial, antiparasitic, neuroprotective, anti-inflammatory, and anticancer activities [176–178]. To the best of our knowledge, natural or synthetic phenazines have not been tested for SCZ, insomnia, or neurodegeneration. Pontemazines A and B are neuroprotective phenazine derivatives that, in animal studies, have rescued hippocampal neurons from glutamate cytotoxicity, highlighting their pro-cognitive properties which could benefit patients with negative symptoms of SCZ or neurodegenerative disorders [176].

Synthetic phenazines exert antioxidant and radical-scavenging properties, and inhibit lipid peroxidation, suggesting beneficial effects in severe insomnia, mental illness and neurodegeneration [179,180] (Figure 3). Moreover, halogenated phenazines act as iron chelators, likely preventing neuronal ferroptosis [181]. We believe that pontemazines and halogenated phenazines should be assessed for antipsychotic/anti-neurodegenerative properties.

From the biochemical standpoint, phenazines are almost identical to phenothiazine antipsychotics and likely possess similar properties (Figure 4). Phenothiazines are typical antipsychotic drugs utilized primarily for SCZ and SLDs, which block dopaminergic transmission at the level of postsynaptic neuron. Several phenothiazines influence other receptors, including adrenergic, histaminergic, and cholinergic, exerting various clinical effects as well as adverse reactions. Aside from psychotic disorders, phenothiazines are also used for the treatment of migraine headaches, hiccups, nausea, vomiting, and cancer [182]. Like phenazines, phenothiazines intercalate themselves into the lipid bilayer of plasma and mitochondrial membranes, disrupting the curvature and receptor alignment on neuronal/mitochondrial surfaces [183] (Figure 3). In contrast, oxidized lipids, including 7-ketocholesterol (7KCl), form looped structures, generating membrane curvatures and pores that may trigger cell death [184].

Antioxidant phenothiazine and their derivatives have recently been developed for cancer, cardiovascular disease (CVD), *Mycobacterium leprae* and other antibiotic-resistant microbes [185,186].

Phenothiazine derivatives exert anti-peroxidation properties and protect against lipid pathology and ferroptosis, suggesting efficacy as antipsychotic drugs [187]. In addition, antioxidant phenothiazines are likely beneficial for insomnia and neurodegenerative disorders, suggesting that these compounds should be tested for neuropsychiatric pathology [186].

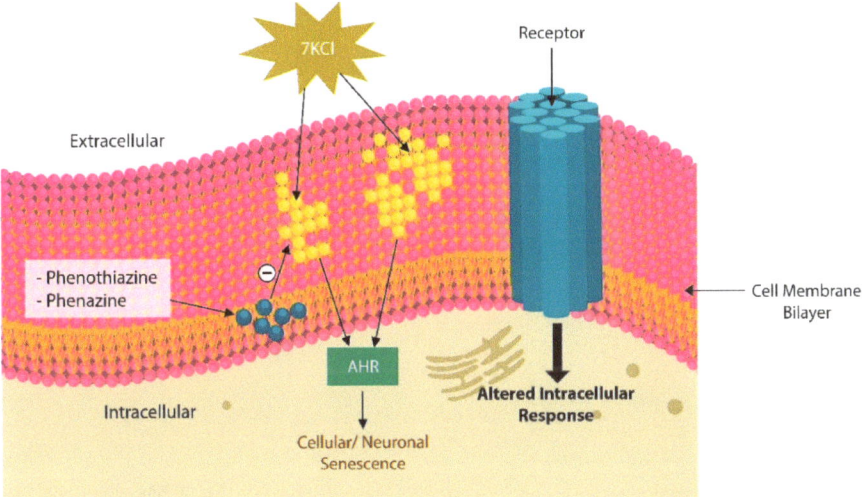

Figure 3. The lipid bilayer of neuronal membrane is easily oxidated when intracellular iron is upregulated. Oxysterols, including 7-Ketocholesterol (a toxic oxide), and oxidated phospholipids alter the biophysical properties of cell membranes, disrupting neurotransmission. In addition, oxidized lipids activate AhR, triggering premature neuronal senescence. Phenazines, phenothiazines, and their derivatives, intercalate themselves into the lipid bilayer, repairing the lipids in cellular and/or mitochondrial membranes.

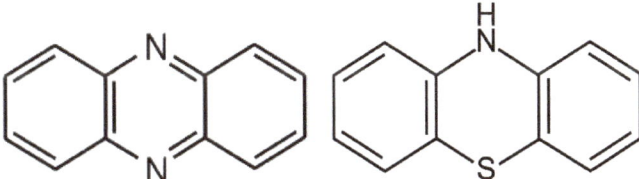

Figure 4. Phenazine vs. phenothiazine: similarities and differences.

Propenylphenothiazine is a potent antioxidant with electron-donor capability that could prevent gray matter loss, a hallmark of SCZ and SLDs [188,189]. Electron-donating psychotropic drugs have been known to preserve the brain volume, suggesting that propenylphenothiazine may treat psychosis without reducing the gray matter volume. The majority of conventional antipsychotic drugs are electron-acceptors which often lower the brain volume as documented by many neuroimaging studies [190]. An even newer category of tetracyclic and pentacyclic phenothiazines with antioxidant properties has recently been developed, suggesting likely efficacy for cognitive impairment and negative SCZ symptoms. Moreover, the N10-carbonyl-substituted phenothiazines were demonstrated to inhibit lipid peroxidation, suggesting superior antipsychotic efficacy [191].

Natural and some synthetic phenazines and novel antioxidant phenothiazines have not been tested for SCZ, insomnia or neurodegenerative disorders but are likely efficient somnogens and antipsychotics. For example, synthetic phenazines, known as pontemazines A and B, rescued hippocampal neurons from glutamate cytotoxicity in rodents, highlighting their pro-cognitive properties which could benefit patients with negative symptoms of SCZ [192].

2.4. Natural Antioxidants

SCZ and SLDs have been associated with premature cellular senescence, a phenotype marked by shortened telomeres, accumulation of macromolecular aggregates, increased level of senescence-associated β-galactosidase (SA-β-gal) and a detrimental secretome known as senescence-associated secretory phenotype (SASP).

Natural Antioxidant Foods

Antioxidants are major players in repairing damages to macromolecules, opposing pathological events associated with cellular senescence (Table 1). Since AhR is the master regulator of cellular senescence and responds to external pollutants (such as polycyclic aromatic hydrocarbons (PAHs) as well as internal toxins, including oxidized lipids, antioxidants likely have the opposite effect.

Table 1. SCZ-relevant antioxidants and sources.

Antioxidants	Source	References
Lycopene	Grape skin, guava, grapefruit, blueberries, tomatoes	[193]
Apigenin	Cabbage, blueberries, acai berries	[194]
Phenolic acid	Oilseeds, cereals, grains	[195]
Curcumin	chicken, beef, tofu, vegetables	[196]
Epigallocatechin gallate	Apples, blackberries, broad beans, cherries, black grapes, pears, raspberries, and chocolate	[197]
Berberine	Oregon grape, phellodendron, and tree turmeric.	[198]
Quercetin	Fruits, apples, onions, parsley, sage, tea, and red wine	[199]
Kempferol	Fruits and vegetables.	[200]
Tocopherols	Oilseed, cereals, eggs, deary products	[201]

2.5. Mitochondrial Transfer and Transplantation

Early studies on mitochondrial transplantation from the 1980s utilized co-incubation of various cell types with naked mitochondria, hoping that cells would internalize the organelles from the extracellular environment [202–204]. Later, HeLa cells and mesenchymal stem cells were used as mitochondrial sources and found that successful organelle uptake occurred in a short time interval of 1–2 h [205–207]. At present, mitochondrial transplantation into cardiomyocytes has been accomplished successfully and confirmed by mitochondrial DNA (mtDNA) detected in host cells [208,209].

Mitochondrial transplantation and neuronal rescue from ferroptosis have been performed successfully in both animals and humans, suggesting a novel strategy for neurometabolic disorders [210]. To our knowledge, mitochondrial transplantation has not been attempted in sleep disorders, while in mental illness, it has been tried in animal models only [132]. Trafficking mitochondria from astrocytes and microglia to neurons can take place spontaneously after brain injuries, reflecting a likely compensatory mechanism to preserve neuronal viability [211]. In addition, it has been established that SSRIs, GJA1-20K, and CD38 signaling can facilitate mitochondrial transfer, emphasizing potential strategies for insomnia, severe mental illness, and neurodegeneration [210,211].

3. Conclusions

Forensic detainees with severe mental illness and comorbid insomnia age at an accelerated pace, suggesting that premature cellular senescence, a characteristic of SCZ, may comprise the common pathway where sleep and mental illness intersect. Loss of neurons due to impaired sleep may trigger the premature development of dementia and other age-related conditions, known to occur earlier in life compared to the general population. These comorbidities increase healthcare expenditures and shorten patients' lifespan; thus, identifying and treating these conditions early is crucial.

YOD, a category of neurodegenerative disorders which include bvFTD, has been on the rise over the past few decades, as evidenced by the increased number of first offenders before the age of 65. Selective loss of VENs in bvFTD is likely due to the large size of these cells, predisposed to peroxidation of plasma membrane lipids and mitochondrial loss by dysfunctional autophagy.

At the molecular level, AhR is the equivalent of VENs, as this protein responds to both endogenous and exogenous ligands, including lipid peroxides and other insomnia and psychosis-related molecules.

Antioxidants and phenazine and phenothiazine derivatives are AhR ligands, highlighting potential natural treatment strategies against psychosis, insomnia, and neurodegeneration.

Author Contributions: Conceptualization, A.S. and P.G.B.; methodology, N.J.; validation, K.A.T. and I.A.O.; writing—review and editing, P.G.B. All authors have read and agreed to the published version of the manuscript.

Funding: This research received no external funding.

Institutional Review Board Statement: Not applicable.

Informed Consent Statement: Not applicable.

Data Availability Statement: Not applicable.

Conflicts of Interest: The authors declare no conflicts of interest.

References

1. Sateia, M.J.; Doghramji, K.; Hauri, P.J.; Morin, C.M. Evaluation of chronic insomnia. An American Academy of Sleep Medicine review. *Sleep* **2000**, *23*, 243–308. [CrossRef]
2. Dewa, L.H.; Thibaut, B.; Pattison, N.; Campbell, S.J.; Woodcock, T.; Aylin, P.; Archer, S. Treating insomnia in people who are incarcerated: A feasibility study of a multi-component treatment pathway. *Sleep Adv.* **2024**, *5*, zpae003. [CrossRef]
3. Talih, F.; Ajaltouni, J.; Ghandour, H.; Abu-Mohammad, A.S.; Kobeissy, F. Insomnia in hospitalized psychiatric patients: Prevalence and associated factors. *Neuropsychiatr. Dis. Treat.* **2018**, *14*, 969–975. [CrossRef]
4. Levichkina, E.V.; Busygina, I.I.; Pigareva, M.L.; Pigarev, I.N. The Mysterious Island: Insula and Its Dual Function in Sleep and Wakefulness. *Front. Syst. Neurosci.* **2021**, *14*, 592660. [CrossRef] [PubMed]
5. Xu, H.; Shen, H.; Wang, L.; Zhong, Q.; Lei, Y.; Yang, L.; Zeng, L.L.; Zhou, Z.; Hu, D.; Yang, Z. Impact of 36 h of total sleep depri-vation on resting-state dynamic functional connectivity. *Brain Res.* **2018**, *1688*, 22–32. [CrossRef] [PubMed]
6. Wylie, K.P.; Tregellas, J.R. The role of the insula in schizophrenia. *Schizophr. Res.* **2010**, *123*, 93–104. [CrossRef] [PubMed]
7. Fathy, Y.Y.; Hoogers, S.E.; Berendse, H.W.; van der Werf, Y.D.; Visser, P.J.; de Jong, F.J.; van de Berg, W.D. Differential insular cortex sub-regional atrophy in neurodegenerative diseases: A systematic review and meta-analysis. *Brain Imaging Behav.* **2019**, *14*, 2799–2816. [CrossRef] [PubMed]
8. Koutsouleris, N.; Pantelis, C.; Velakoulis, D.; McGuire, P.; Dwyer, D.B.; Urquijo-Castro, M.-F.; Paul, R.; Dong, S.; Popovic, D.; Oeztuerk, O.; et al. Exploring Links Between Psychosis and Frontotemporal Dementia Using Multimodal Machine Learning: Dementia Praecox Revisited. *JAMA Psychiatry* **2022**, *79*, 907–919. [CrossRef]
9. Triarhou, L.C. The percipient observations of Constantin von Economo on encephalitis lethargica and sleep disruption and their lasting impact on contemporary sleep research. *Brain Res. Bull.* **2006**, *69*, 244–258. [CrossRef]
10. Allman, J.M.; Tetreault, N.A.; Hakeem, A.Y.; Manaye, K.F.; Semendeferi, K.; Erwin, J.M.; Park, S.; Goubert, V.; Hof, P.R. The von Economo neurons in frontoinsular and anterior cingulate cortex in great apes and humans. *Brain Struct. Funct.* **2010**, *214*, 495–517. [CrossRef]
11. Berg, M.T.; Rogers, E.M.; Lei, M.-K.; Simons, R.L. Losing Years Doing Time: Incarceration Exposure and Accelerated Biological Aging among African American Adults. *J. Health Soc. Behav.* **2021**, *62*, 460–476. [CrossRef]
12. Kaiksow, F.A.; Brown, L.; Merss, K.B. Caring for the Rapidly Aging Incarcerated Population: The Role of Policy. *J. Gerontol. Nurs.* **2023**, *49*, 7–11. [CrossRef] [PubMed]
13. Papanastasiou, E.; Gaughran, F.; Smith, S. Schizophrenia as segmental progeria. *J. R. Soc. Med.* **2011**, *104*, 475–484. [CrossRef] [PubMed]
14. Killilea, D.W.; Wong, S.L.; Cahaya, H.S.; Atamna, H.; Ames, B.N. Iron accumulation during cellular senescence. *Ann. N. Y. Acad. Sci.* **2004**, *1019*, 365–367. [CrossRef] [PubMed]
15. Urrutia, P.J.; Mena, N.P.; Núñez, M.T. The interplay between iron accumulation, mitochondrial dysfunction, and inflammation during the execution step of neurodegenerative disorders. *Front. Pharmacol.* **2014**, *5*, 38. [CrossRef] [PubMed]

16. Carvalhas-Almeida, C.; Cavadas, C.; Álvaro, A.R. The impact of insomnia on frailty and the hallmarks of aging. *Aging Clin. Exp. Res.* **2022**, *35*, 253–269. [CrossRef] [PubMed]
17. Carroll, J.E.; Prather, A.A. Sleep and biological aging: A short review. *Curr. Opin. Endocr. Metab. Res.* **2021**, *18*, 159–164. [CrossRef] [PubMed]
18. Skonieczna-Żydecka, K.; Jamioł-Milc, D.; Borecki, K.; Stachowska, E.; Zabielska, P.; Kamińska, M.; Karakiewicz, B. The Prevalence of Insomnia and the Link between Iron Metabolism Genes Polymorphisms, TF rs1049296 C>T, TF rs3811647 G>A, TFR rs7385804 A>C, HAMP rs10421768 A>G and Sleep Disorders in Polish Individuals with ASD. *Int. J. Environ. Res. Public Health* **2020**, *17*, 400 [CrossRef]
19. Nacarino-Palma, A.; Rico-Leo, E.M.; Campisi, J.; Ramanathan, A.; González-Rico, F.J.; Rejano-Gordillo, C.M.; Ordiales-Talavero, A.; Merino, J.M.; Fernández-Salguero, P.M. Aryl hydrocarbon receptor blocks aging-induced senescence in the liver and fibroblast cells. *Aging* **2022**, *14*, 4281–4304. [CrossRef]
20. Panda, S.K.; Peng, V.; Sudan, R.; Antonova, A.U.; Di Luccia, B.; Ohara, T.E.; Fachi, J.L.; Grajales-Reyes, G.E.; Jaeger, N.; Trsan, T.; et al. Repression of the aryl-hydrocarbon receptor prevents oxidative stress and ferroptosis of intestinal intraepithelial lymphocytes. *Immunity* **2023**, *56*, 797–812.e4. [CrossRef]
21. Hwang, H.J.; Dornbos, P.; Steidemann, M.; Dunivin, T.K.; Rizzo, M.; LaPres, J.J. Mitochondrial-targeted aryl hydrocarbon receptor and the impact of 2,3,7,8-tetrachlorodibenzo-p-dioxin on cellular respiration and the mitochondrial proteome. *Toxicol. Appl. Pharmacol.* **2016**, *304*, 121–132. [CrossRef]
22. Dietrich-Muszalska, A.; Kontek, B. Lipid peroxidation in patients with schizophrenia. *Psychiatry Clin. Neurosci.* **2010**, *64*, 469–475. [CrossRef] [PubMed]
23. Feng, S.; Chen, J.; Qu, C.; Yang, L.; Wu, X.; Wang, S.; Yang, T.; Liu, H.; Fang, Y.; Sun, P. Identification of Ferroptosis-Related Genes in Schizophrenia Based on Bioinformatic Analysis. *Genes* **2022**, *13*, 2168. [CrossRef] [PubMed]
24. Gulec, M.; Ozkol, H.; Selvi, Y.; Tuluce, Y.; Aydin, A.; Besiroglu, L.; Ozdemir, P.G. Oxidative stress in patients with primary insomnia. *Prog. Neuro-Psychopharmacol. Biol. Psychiatry* **2012**, *37*, 247–251. [CrossRef]
25. Liang, H.; Van Remmen, H.; Frohlich, V.; Lechleiter, J.; Richardson, A.; Ran, Q. Gpx4 protects mitochondrial ATP generation against oxidative damage. *Biochem. Biophys. Res. Commun.* **2007**, *356*, 893–898. [CrossRef]
26. Seibt, T.M.; Proneth, B.; Conrad, M. Role of GPX4 in ferroptosis and its pharmacological implication. *Free Radic. Biol. Med.* **2018**, *133*, 144–152. [CrossRef] [PubMed]
27. Azuma, K.; Koumura, T.; Iwamoto, R.; Matsuoka, M.; Terauchi, R.; Yasuda, S.; Shiraya, T.; Watanabe, S.; Aihara, M.; Imai, H.; et al. Mitochondrial glutathione peroxidase 4 is indispensable for photoreceptor development and survival in mice. *J. Biol. Chem.* **2022**, *298*, 101824. [CrossRef] [PubMed]
28. Dixon, S.J.; Lemberg, K.M.; Lamprecht, M.R.; Skouta, R.; Zaitsev, E.M.; Gleason, C.E.; Patel, D.N.; Bauer, A.J.; Cantley, A.M.; Yang, W.S.; et al. Fer-roptosis: An iron-dependent form of nonapoptotic cell death. *Cell* **2012**, *149*, 1060–1072. [CrossRef]
29. Miwa, S.; Kashyap, S.; Chini, E.; von Zglinicki, T. Mitochondrial dysfunction in cell senescence and aging. *J. Clin. Investig.* **2022**, *132*, e158447. [CrossRef]
30. Carroll, J.E.; Esquivel, S.; Goldberg, A.; Seeman, T.E.; Effros, R.B.; Dock, J.; Olmstead, R.; Breen, E.C.; Irwin, M.R. Insomnia and Telomere Length in Older Adults. *Sleep* **2016**, *39*, 559–564. [CrossRef]
31. Schnack, H.G.; van Haren, N.E.; Nieuwenhuis, M.; Hulshoff Pol, H.E.; Cahn, W.; Kahn, R.S. Accelerated Brain Aging in Schizophrenia: A Longitudinal Pattern Recognition Study. *Am. J. Psychiatry* **2016**, *173*, 607–616. [CrossRef]
32. Porterfield, V.; Khan, S.S.; Foff, E.P.; Koseoglu, M.M.; Blanco, I.K.; Jayaraman, S.; Lien, E.; McConnell, M.J.; Bloom, G.S.; Lazo, J.S.; et al. A three-dimensional dementia model reveals spontaneous cell cycle re-entry and a senescence-associated secretory phenotype. *Neurobiol. Aging* **2020**, *90*, 125–134. [CrossRef]
33. De Lorenzo, B.H.; Marchioro, L.d.O.; Greco, C.R.; Suchecki, D. Sleep-deprivation reduces NK cell number and function mediated by β-adrenergic signalling. *Psychoneuroendocrinology* **2015**, *57*, 134–143. [CrossRef] [PubMed]
34. Tarantino, N.; Leboyer, M.; Bouleau, A.; Hamdani, N.; Richard, J.R.; Boukouaci, W.; Ching-Lien, W.; Godin, O.; Bengoufa, D.; Le Corvoisier, P.; et al. Natural killer cells in first-episode psychosis: An innate immune signature? *Mol. Psychiatry* **2021**, *26*, 5297–5306. [CrossRef]
35. Huang, A.; Shinde, P.V.; Huang, J.; Senff, T.; Xu, H.C.; Margotta, C.; Häussinger, D.; Willnow, T.E.; Zhang, J.; Pandyra, A.A.; et al. Progranulin prevents regulatory NK cell cytotoxicity against antiviral T cells. *J. Clin. Investig.* **2019**, *4*, e129856. [CrossRef] [PubMed]
36. Irwin, M.R. Sleep disruption induces activation of inflammation and heightens risk for infectious disease: Role of impairments in thermoregulation and elevated ambient temperature. *Temperature* **2022**, *10*, 198–234. [CrossRef]
37. Bright, F.; Werry, E.L.; Dobson-Stone, C.; Piguet, O.; Ittner, L.M.; Halliday, G.M.; Hodges, J.R.; Kiernan, M.C.; Loy, C.T.; Kassiou, M.; et al. Neuroinflammation in frontotemporal dementia. *Nat. Rev. Neurol.* **2019**, *15*, 540–555. [CrossRef]
38. Vallée, A. Neuroinflammation in Schizophrenia: The Key Role of the WNT/β-Catenin Pathway. *Int. J. Mol. Sci.* **2022**, *23*, 2810. [CrossRef]
39. Nesci, S.; Spagnoletta, A.; Oppedisano, F. Inflammation, Mitochondria and Natural Compounds Together in the Circle of Trust. *Int. J. Mol. Sci.* **2023**, *24*, 6106. [CrossRef] [PubMed]
40. Andrieux, P.; Chevillard, C.; Cunha-Neto, E.; Nunes, J.P.S. Mitochondria as a Cellular Hub in Infection and Inflammation. *Int. J Mol. Sci.* **2021**, *22*, 11338. [CrossRef]

41. Hayakawa, K.; Esposito, E.; Wang, X.; Terasaki, Y.; Liu, Y.; Xing, C.; Ji, X.; Lo, E.H. Transfer of mitochondria from astrocytes to neurons after stroke. *Nature* **2016**, *535*, 551–555. [CrossRef]
42. Gollihue, J.; Norris, C. Astrocyte mitochondria: Central players and potential therapeutic targets for neurodegenerative diseases and injury. *Ageing Res. Rev.* **2020**, *59*, 101039. [CrossRef] [PubMed]
43. Boas, S.M.; Joyce, K.L.; Cowell, R.M. The NRF2-Dependent Transcriptional Regulation of Antioxidant Defense Pathways: Relevance for Cell Type-Specific Vulnerability to Neurodegeneration and Therapeutic Intervention. *Antioxidants* **2021**, *11*, 8. [CrossRef] [PubMed]
44. Downar, J.; Crawley, A.P.; Mikulis, D.J.; Davis, K.D. A multimodal cortical network for the detection of changes in the sensory environment. *Nat. Neurosci.* **2000**, *3*, 277–283. [CrossRef] [PubMed]
45. Wolff, M.; Vann, S.D. The cognitive thalamus as a gateway to mental representations. *J. Neurosci.* **2018**, *39*, 3–14. [CrossRef]
46. Sridharan, D.; Levitin, D.J.; Menon, V. A critical role for the right fronto-insular cortex in switching between central-executive and default-mode networks. *Proc. Natl. Acad. Sci. USA* **2008**, *105*, 12569–12574. [CrossRef]
47. Ueno, D.; Matsuoka, T.; Kato, Y.; Ayani, N.; Maeda, S.; Takeda, M.; Narumoto, J. Individual Differences in Interoceptive Accuracy Are Correlated with Salience Network Connectivity in Older Adults. *Front. Aging Neurosci.* **2020**, *12*, 592002. [CrossRef]
48. Blessing, W.W.; Blessing, E.M.; Mohammed, M.; Ootsuka, Y. Clozapine, chlorpromazine and risperidone dose-dependently reduce emotional hyperthermia, a biological marker of salience. *Psychopharmacology* **2017**, *234*, 3259–3269. [CrossRef]
49. Seeley, W.W. The Salience Network: A Neural System for Perceiving and Responding to Homeostatic Demands. *J. Neurosci.* **2019**, *39*, 9878–9882. [CrossRef] [PubMed]
50. Pasquini, L.; Nana, A.L.; Toller, G.; Brown, J.A.; Deng, J.; Staffaroni, A.; Kim, E.-J.; Hwang, J.-H.L.; Li, L.; Park, Y.; et al. Salience Network Atrophy Links Neuron Type-Specific Pathobiology to Loss of Empathy in Frontotemporal Dementia. *Cereb. Cortex* **2020**, *30*, 5387–5399. [CrossRef] [PubMed]
51. Mendez, M.F.; Anderson, E.; Shapira, J.S. An investigate von of moral judgement in frontotemporal dementia. *Cogn. Behav. Neurol.* **2005**, *18*, 193–197. [CrossRef]
52. Mendez, M.F. The neurobiology of moral behavior: Review and neuropsychiatric implications. *CNS Spectr.* **2009**, *14*, 608–620. [CrossRef] [PubMed]
53. Boeve, B.F. Behavioral Variant Frontotemporal Dementia. *Continuum* **2022**, *28*, 702–725. [CrossRef] [PubMed]
54. Arrigoni, E.; Fuller, P.M. The Sleep-Promoting Ventrolateral Preoptic Nucleus: What Have We Learned over the Past 25 Years? *Int. J. Mol. Sci.* **2022**, *23*, 2905. [CrossRef] [PubMed]
55. De Luca, R.; Nardone, S.; Grace, K.P.; Venner, A.; Cristofolini, M.; Bandaru, S.S.; Sohn, L.T.; Kong, D.; Mochizuki, T.; Viberti, B.; et al. Orexin neurons inhibit sleep to promote arousal. *Nat. Commun.* **2022**, *13*, 4163. [CrossRef] [PubMed]
56. Inutsuka, A.; Yamanaka, A. The regulation of sleep and wakefulness by the hypothalamic neuropeptide orexin/hypocretin. *Nagoya J. Med. Sci.* **2013**, *75*, 29–36.
57. Yin, D.; Dong, H.; Wang, T.-X.; Hu, Z.-Z.; Cheng, N.-N.; Qu, W.-M.; Huang, Z.-L. Glutamate Activates the Histaminergic Tuberomammillary Nucleus and Increases Wakefulness in Rats. *Neuroscience* **2019**, *413*, 86–98. [CrossRef] [PubMed]
58. Konadhode, R.R.; Pelluru, D.; Shiromani, P.J. Neurons containing orexin or melanin concentrating hormone reciprocally regulate wake and sleep. *Front. Syst. Neurosci.* **2015**, *8*, 244. [CrossRef]
59. Chung, S.; Weber, F.; Zhong, P.; Tan, C.L.; Nguyen, T.N.; Beier, K.T.; Hörmann, N.; Chang, W.-C.; Zhang, Z.; Do, J.P.; et al. Identification of preoptic sleep neurons using retrograde labelling and gene profiling. *Nature* **2017**, *545*, 477–481. [CrossRef]
60. Bandarabadi, M.; Li, S.; Aeschlimann, L.; Colombo, G.; Tzanoulinou, S.; Tafti, M.; Becchetti, A.; Boutrel, B.; Vassalli, A. Inactivation of hypocretin receptor-2 signaling in dopaminergic neurons induces hyperarousal and enhanced cognition but impaired inhibitory control. *Mol. Psychiatry* **2023**. online ahead of print. [CrossRef]
61. Wu, S.; Gao, C.; Han, F.; Cheng, H. Histamine H1 receptor in basal forebrain cholinergic circuit: A novel target for the negative symptoms of schizophrenia? *Neurosci. Bull.* **2022**, *38*, 558–560. [CrossRef]
62. Grady, F.S.; Boes, A.D.; Geerling, J.C. A Century Searching for the Neurons Necessary for Wakefulness. *Front. Neurosci.* **2022**, *16*, 930514. [CrossRef]
63. Kerkhofs, M.; Lavie, P. Frédéric Bremer 1892–1982: A pioneer in sleep research. *Sleep Med. Rev.* **2000**, *4*, 505–514. [CrossRef]
64. Fuller, P.; Sherman, D.; Pedersen, N.P.; Saper, C.B.; Lu, J. Reassessment of the structural basis of the ascending arousal system. *J. Comp. Neurol.* **2010**, *519*, 933–956, Erratum in *J. Comp. Neurol.* **2011**, *519*, 3817. [CrossRef] [PubMed]
65. Lavie, P. The sleep theory of Constantin von Economo. *J. Sleep Res.* **1993**, *2*, 175–178. [CrossRef]
66. Vyas, A.; De Jesus, O. Von Economo Encephalitis. In *StatPearls [Internet]*; StatPearls Publishing: Treasure Island, FL, USA, 2024.
67. Rosen, D. Asleep: The Forgotten Epidemic That Remains One of Medicine's Greatest Mysteries. *J. Clin. Sleep Med.* **2010**, *6*, 299. [CrossRef]
68. Cortelli, P.; Perani, D.; Parchi, P.; Grassi, F.; Montagna, P.; De Martin, M.; Castellani, R.; Tinuper, P.; Gambetti, P.; Lugaresi, E.; et al. Cerebral metabolism in fatal familial insomnia: Relation to duration, neuropathology, and distribution of protease-resistent prion protein. *Neurology* **1997**, *49*, 126–133. [CrossRef]
69. Gallassi, R.; Morreale, A.; Montagna, P.; Cortelli, P.; Avoni, P.; Castellani, R.; Gambetti, R.; Lugaresi, E. Fatal familial insomnia: Behavioral and cognitive features. *Neurology* **1996**, *46*, 935–939. [CrossRef] [PubMed]

70. Sturm, V.E.; Brown, J.A.; Hua, A.Y.; Lwi, S.J.; Zhou, J.; Kurth, F.; Eickhoff, S.B.; Rosen, H.J.; Kramer, J.H.; Miller, B.L.; et al. Network Architecture Underlying Basal Autonomic Outflow: Evidence from Frontotemporal Dementia. *J. Neurosci.* **2018**, *38*, 8943–8955. [CrossRef] [PubMed]
71. Mallikarjun, P.K.; Lalousis, P.A.; Dunne, T.F.; Heinze, K.; Reniers, R.L.; Broome, M.R.; Farmah, B.; Oyebode, F.; Wood, S.J.; Upthegrove, R. Aberrant salience network functional connectivity in auditory verbal hallucinations: A first episode psychosis sample. *Transl. Psychiatry* **2018**, *8*, 69. [CrossRef] [PubMed]
72. Cracco, L.; Appleby, B.S.; Gambetti, P. Fatal familial insomnia and sporadic fatal insomnia. In *Handbook of Clinical Neurology*; Elsevier: Amsterdam, The Netherlands, 2018; Volume 153, pp. 271–299. [CrossRef]
73. Wang, Y.; Li, M.; Li, W.; Xiao, L.; Huo, X.; Ding, J.; Sun, T. Is the insula linked to sleep? A systematic review and narrative synthesis. *Heliyon* **2022**, *8*, e11406. [CrossRef]
74. Hehr, A.; Huntley, E.D.; Marusak, H.A. Getting a Good Night's Sleep: Associations Between Sleep Duration and Par-ent-Reported Sleep Quality on Default Mode Network Connectivity in Youth. *J. Adolesc. Health* **2023**, *72*, 933–942. [CrossRef] [PubMed]
75. Guo, Y.; Zou, G.; Shao, Y.; Chen, J.; Li, Y.; Liu, J.; Yao, P.; Zhou, S.; Xu, J.; Hu, S.; et al. Increased connectivity of the anterior cingulate cortex is associated with the tendency to awakening during N2 sleep in patients with insomnia disorder. *Sleep* **2022**, *46*, zsac290. [CrossRef] [PubMed]
76. Guldenmund, P.; Demertzi, A.; Boveroux, P.; Boly, M.; Vanhaudenhuyse, A.; Bruno, M.-A.; Gosseries, O.; Noirhomme, Q.; Brichant, J.-F.; Bonhomme, V.; et al. Thalamus, brainstem and salience network connectivity changes during propofol-induced sedation and unconsciousness. *Brain Connect.* **2013**, *3*, 273–285. [CrossRef] [PubMed]
77. Zhang, L.; Luo, L.; Zhou, Z.; Xu, K.; Zhang, L.; Liu, X.; Tan, X.; Zhang, J.; Ye, X.; Gao, J.; et al. Functional Connectivity of Anterior Insula Predicts Recovery of Patients with Disorders of Consciousness. *Front. Neurol.* **2018**, *9*, 1024. [CrossRef]
78. Mashour, G.A. Anesthetizing the Self: The Neurobiology of Humbug. *Anesthesiology* **2016**, *124*, 747–749. [CrossRef] [PubMed]
79. Qi, J.; Li, B.-Z.; Zhang, Y.; Pan, B.; Gao, Y.-H.; Zhan, H.; Liu, Y.; Shao, Y.-C.; Zhang, X. Altered insula-prefrontal functional connectivity correlates to decreased vigilant attention after total sleep deprivation. *Sleep Med.* **2021**, *84*, 187–194. [CrossRef]
80. Li, C.; Dong, M.; Yin, Y.; Hua, K.; Fu, S.; Jiang, G. Aberrant Effective Connectivity of the Right Anterior Insula in Primary Insomnia. *Front. Neurol.* **2018**, *9*, 317. [CrossRef]
81. Chen, M.C.; Chiang, W.-Y.; Yugay, T.; Patxot, M.; Ozcivit, I.B.; Hu, K.; Lu, J. Anterior Insula Regulates Multiscale Temporal Organization of Sleep and Wake Activity. *J. Biol. Rhythm.* **2016**, *31*, 182–193. [CrossRef]
82. Palaniyappan, L.; White, T.; Liddle, P. The concept of salience network dysfunction in schizophrenia: From neuroimaging observations to therapeutic opportunities. *Curr. Top. Med. Chem.* **2012**, *12*, 2324–2338. [CrossRef]
83. Huang, H.; Chen, C.; Rong, B.; Wan, Q.; Chen, J.; Liu, Z.; Zhou, Y.; Wang, G.; Wang, H. Resting-state functional connectivity of salience network in schizophrenia and depression. *Sci. Rep.* **2022**, *12*, 11204. [CrossRef]
84. He, X.; Qin, W.; Liu, Y.; Zhang, X.; Duan, Y.; Song, J.; Li, K.; Jiang, T.; Yu, C. Abnormal salience network in normal aging and in amnestic mild cognitive impairment and Alzheimer's disease. *Hum. Brain Mapp.* **2013**, *35*, 3446–3464. [CrossRef] [PubMed]
85. Putcha, D.; Ross, R.S.; Cronin-Golomb, A.; Janes, A.C.; Stern, C.E. Salience and Default Mode Network Coupling Predicts Cognition in Aging and Parkinson's Disease. *J. Int. Neuropsychol. Soc.* **2016**, *22*, 205–215. [CrossRef] [PubMed]
86. Day, G.S.; Farb, N.A.S.; Tang-Wai, D.F.; Masellis, M.; Black, S.E.; Freedman, M.; Pollock, B.G.; Chow, T.W. Salience Network Resting-State Activity: Prediction of Frontotemporal Dementia Pro-gression. *JAMA Neurol.* **2013**, *70*, 1249–1253. [CrossRef] [PubMed]
87. Sheffield, J.M.; Rogers, B.P.; Blackford, J.U.; Heckers, S.; Woodward, N.D. Insula functional connectivity in schizophrenia. *Schizophr. Res.* **2020**, *220*, 69–77. [CrossRef]
88. Adams, R.; David, A.S. Patterns of anterior cingulate activation in schizophrenia: A selective review. *Neuropsychiatr. Dis. Treat.* **2007**, *3*, 87–101. [CrossRef]
89. Nana, A.L.; Sidhu, M.; Gaus, S.E.; Hwang, J.-H.L.; Li, L.; Park, Y.; Kim, E.-J.; Pasquini, L.; Allen, I.E.; Rankin, K.P.; et al. Neurons selectively targeted in frontotemporal dementia reveal early stage TDP-43 pathobiology. *Acta Neuropathol.* **2018**, *137*, 27–46. [CrossRef] [PubMed]
90. Zago, S.; Scarpazza, C.; Difonzo, T.; Arighi, A.; Hajhajate, D.; Torrente, Y.; Sartori, G. Behavioral Variant of Frontotemporal Dementia and Homicide in a Historical Case. *J. Am. Acad. Psychiatry Law* **2021**, *49*, 219–227. [PubMed]
91. Nilsson, C.; Waldö, M.L.; Nilsson, K.; Santillo, A.; Vestberg, S. Age-related incidence and family history in frontotemporal dementia: Data from the swedish dementia registry. *PLoS ONE* **2014**, *9*, e94901. [CrossRef]
92. Hendriks, S.; Peetoom, K.; Bakker, C.; van der Flier, W.M.; Papma, J.M.; Koopmans, R.; Verhey, F.R.J.; de Vugt, M.; Köhler, S.; Withall, A.; et al. Global Prevalence of Young-Onset Dementia: A Systematic Review and Meta-analysis. *JAMA Neurol.* **2021**, *78*, 1080–1090. [CrossRef]
93. Onyike, C.U.; Diehl-Schmid, J. The epidemiology of frontotemporal dementia. *Int. Rev. Psychiatry* **2013**, *25*, 130–137. [CrossRef]
94. Diehl-Schmid, J.; Perneczky, R.; Koch, J.; Nedopil, N.; Kurz, A. Guilty by suspicion? Criminal behavior in frontotemporal lobar degeneration. *Cogn. Behav. Neurol.* **2013**, *26*, 73–77. [CrossRef]
95. Krause, M.; Theiss, C.; Brüne, M. Ultrastructural Alterations of Von Economo Neurons in the Anterior Cingulate Cortex in Schizophrenia. *Anat. Rec.* **2017**, *300*, 2017–2024. [CrossRef]
96. Kim, S.H.; Kim, Y.J.; Lee, B.H.; Lee, P.; Park, J.H.; Seo, S.W.; Jeong, Y. Behavioral Reserve in Behavioral Variant Frontotemporal Dementia. *Front. Aging Neurosci.* **2022**, *14*, 875589. [CrossRef]

97. Vohryzek, J.; Cabral, J.; Vuust, P.; Deco, G.; Kringelbach, M.L. Understanding brain states across spacetime informed by whole-brain modelling. *Philos. Trans. R. Soc. A Math. Phys. Eng. Sci.* **2022**, *380*, 20210247. [CrossRef]
98. Nathani, M.; Jaleel, V.; Turner, A.; Dirvonas, C.; Suryadevara, U.; Tandon, R. When you hear hoofbeats, think horses and zebras: The importance of a wide differential when it comes to frontotemporal lobar degeneration. *Asian J. Psychiatry* **2019**, *47*, 101875. [CrossRef] [PubMed]
99. Herbert, B.M.; Herbert, C.; Pollatos, O. On the Relationship Between Interoceptive Awareness and Alexithymia: Is Interoceptive Awareness Related to Emotional Awareness? *J. Personal.* **2011**, *79*, 1149–1175. [CrossRef]
100. Quadt, L.; Critchley, H.D.; Garfinkel, S.N. The neurobiology of interoception in health and disease. *Ann. N. Y. Acad. Sci.* **2018**, *1428*, 112–128. [CrossRef] [PubMed]
101. Cauda, F.; Geminiani, G.C.; Vercelli, A. Evolutionary appearance of von Economo's neurons in the mammalian cerebral cortex. *Front. Hum. Neurosci.* **2014**, *8*, 104. [CrossRef] [PubMed]
102. Menon, V.; Uddin, L.Q. Saliency, switching, attention and control: A network model of insula function. *Brain Struct. Funct.* **2010**, *214*, 655–667. [CrossRef]
103. López-Ojeda, W.; Hurley, R.A. Von Economo Neuron Involvement in Social Cognitive and Emotional Impairments in Neuropsychiatric Disorders. *J. Neuropsychiatry Clin. Neurosci.* **2022**, *34*, 302–306. [CrossRef]
104. Hodge, R.D.; Miller, J.A.; Novotny, M.; Kalmbach, B.E.; Ting, J.T.; Bakken, T.E.; Aevermann, B.D.; Barkan, E.R.; Berkowitz-Cerasano, M.L.; Cobbs, C.; et al. Transcriptomic evidence that von Economo neurons are regionally specialized extratelencephalic-projecting excitatory neurons. *Nat. Commun.* **2020**, *11*, 1172. [CrossRef] [PubMed]
105. Dijkstra, A.A.; Lin, L.-C.; Nana, A.L.; Gaus, S.E.; Seeley, W.W. Von Economo Neurons and Fork Cells: A Neurochemical Signature Linked to Monoaminergic Function. *Cereb. Cortex* **2016**, *28*, 131–144. [CrossRef] [PubMed]
106. Azizi, S.A. Monoamines: Dopamine, Norepinephrine, and Serotonin, Beyond Modulation, "Switches" That Alter the State of Target Networks. *Neuroscientist* **2020**, *28*, 121–143. [CrossRef] [PubMed]
107. Valli, M.; Cho, S.S.; Uribe, C.; Masellis, M.; Chen, R.; Mihaescu, A.; Strafella, A.P. VMAT2 availability in Parkinson's disease with probable REM sleep behaviour disorder. *Mol. Brain* **2021**, *14*, 165. [CrossRef] [PubMed]
108. Broese, M.; Riemann, D.; Hein, L.; Nissen, C. α-Adrenergic Receptor Function, Arousal and Sleep: Mechanisms and Therapeutic Implications. *Pharmacopsychiatry* **2012**, *45*, 209–216. [CrossRef] [PubMed]
109. Gaus, R.; Popal, M.; Heinsen, H.; Schmitt, A.; Falkai, P.; Hof, P.R.; Schmitz, C.; Vollhardt, A. Reduced cortical neuron number and neuron density in schizophrenia with focus on area 24: A post-mortem case–control study. *Eur. Arch. Psychiatry Clin. Neurosci.* **2022**, *273*, 1209–1223. [CrossRef] [PubMed]
110. Sjögren, M.; Minthon, L.; Passant, U.; Blennow, K.; Wallin, A. Decreased monoamine metabolites in frontotemporal dementia and Alzheimer's disease. *Neurobiol. Aging* **1998**, *19*, 379–384. [CrossRef]
111. Levenson, J.C.; Kay, D.B.; Buysse, D.J. The Pathophysiology of Insomnia. *Chest* **2015**, *147*, 1179–1192. [CrossRef]
112. Zhou, M.; Kiyoshi, C.M. Astrocyte syncytium: A functional reticular system in the brain. *Neural Regen. Res.* **2019**, *14*, 595–596. [CrossRef]
113. Garofalo, S.; Picard, K.; Limatola, C.; Nadjar, A.; Pascual, O.; Tremblay, M.E. Role of Glia in the Regulation of Sleep in Health and Disease. *Compr. Physiol.* **2020**, *10*, 687–712. [CrossRef] [PubMed]
114. Que, M.; Li, Y.; Wang, X.; Zhan, G.; Luo, X.; Zhou, Z. Role of astrocytes in sleep deprivation: Accomplices, resisters, or bystanders? *Front. Cell. Neurosci.* **2023**, *17*, 1188306. [CrossRef] [PubMed]
115. Mader, S.; Brimberg, L. Aquaporin-4 Water Channel in the Brain and Its Implication for Health and Disease. *Cells* **2019**, *8*, 90. [CrossRef] [PubMed]
116. Jessen, N.A.; Munk, A.S.F.; Lundgaard, I.; Nedergaard, M. The Glymphatic System: A Beginner's Guide. *Neurochem. Res.* **2015**, *40*, 2583–2599. [CrossRef] [PubMed]
117. Valenti, D.; Vacca, R.A.; Moro, L.; Atlante, A. Mitochondria Can Cross Cell Boundaries: An Overview of the Biological Relevance, Pathophysiological Implications and Therapeutic Perspectives of Intercellular Mitochondrial Transfer. *Int. J. Mol. Sci.* **2021**, *22*, 8312. [CrossRef] [PubMed]
118. Leow, D.M.-K.; Cheah, I.K.-M.; Fong, Z.W.-J.; Halliwell, B.; Ong, W.-Y. Protective Effect of Ergothioneine against 7-Ketocholesterol-Induced Mitochondrial Damage in hCMEC/D3 Human Brain Endothelial Cells. *Int. J. Mol. Sci.* **2023**, *24*, 5498. [CrossRef] [PubMed]
119. Asami, T.; Bouix, S.; Whitford, T.J.; Shenton, M.E.; Salisbury, D.F.; McCarley, R.W. Longitudinal loss of gray matter volume in patients with first-episode schizophrenia: DARTEL automated analysis and ROI validation. *Neuroimage* **2012**, *59*, 986–996. [CrossRef]
120. Hill, V.M.; O'connor, R.M.; Sissoko, G.B.; Irobunda, I.S.; Leong, S.; Canman, J.C.; Stavropoulos, N.; Shirasu-Hiza, M. A bidirectional relationship between sleep and oxidative stress in Drosophila. *PLoS Biol.* **2018**, *16*, e2005206. [CrossRef]
121. Patergnani, S.; Bonora, M.; Ingusci, S.; Previati, M.; Marchi, S.; Zucchini, S.; Perrone, M.; Wieckowski, M.R.; Castellazzi, M.; Pugliatti, M.; et al. Antipsychotic drugs counteract autophagy and mitophagy in multiple sclerosis. *Proc. Natl. Acad. Sci. USA* **2021**, *118*, e2020078118. [CrossRef]
122. Hirata, Y.; Cai, R.; Volchuk, A.; Steinberg, B.E.; Saito, Y.; Matsuzawa, A.; Grinstein, S.; Freeman, S.A. Lipid peroxidation increases membrane tension, Piezo1 gating, and cation permeability to execute ferroptosis. *Curr. Biol.* **2023**, *33*, 1282–1294.e5. [CrossRef]
123. Heckers, S.; Konradi, C. Hippocampal neurons in schizophrenia. *J. Neural Transm.* **2002**, *109*, 891–905. [CrossRef] [PubMed]

124. Padurariu, M.; Ciobica, A.; Mavroudis, I.; Fotiou, D.; Baloyannis, S. Hippocampal neuronal loss in the CA1 and CA3 areas of Alz-heimer's disease patients. *Psychiatr. Danub.* **2012**, *24*, 152–158. [PubMed]
125. Zhang, P.; Li, Y.-X.; Zhang, Z.-Z.; Yang, Y.; Rao, J.-X.; Xia, L.; Li, X.-Y.; Chen, G.-H.; Wang, F. Astroglial Mechanisms Underlying Chronic Insomnia Disorder: A Clinical Study. *Nat. Sci. Sleep* **2020**, *12*, 693–704. [CrossRef]
126. Bellesi, M.; de Vivo, L.; Chini, M.; Gilli, F.; Tononi, G.; Cirelli, C. Sleep Loss Promotes Astrocytic Phagocytosis and Microglial Activation in Mouse Cerebral Cortex. *J. Neurosci.* **2017**, *37*, 5263–5273. [CrossRef]
127. Vilalta, A.; Brown, G.C. Neurophagy, the phagocytosis of live neurons and synapses by glia, contributes to brain development and disease. *FEBS J.* **2017**, *285*, 3566–3575. [CrossRef] [PubMed]
128. Liddelow, S.A.; Guttenplan, K.A.; Clarke, L.E.; Bennett, F.C.; Bohlen, C.J.; Schirmer, L.; Bennett, M.L.; Münch, A.E.; Chung, W.-S.; Peterson, T.C.; et al. Neurotoxic reactive astrocytes are induced by activated microglia. *Nature* **2017**, *541*, 481–487. [CrossRef]
129. Whitehurst, T.; Howes, O. The role of mitochondria in the pathophysiology of schizophrenia: A critical review of the evidence focusing on mitochondrial complex one. *Neurosci. Biobehav. Rev.* **2021**, *132*, 449–464. [CrossRef]
130. Beaupre, L.M.M.; Brown, G.M.; Braganza, N.A.; Kennedy, J.L.; Gonçalves, V.F. Mitochondria's role in sleep: Novel insights from sleep deprivation and restriction studies. *World J. Biol. Psychiatry* **2021**, *23*, 1–13. [CrossRef]
131. Richardson, R.B.; Mailloux, R.J. Mitochondria Need Their Sleep: Redox, Bioenergetics, and Temperature Regulation of Circadian Rhythms and the Role of Cysteine-Mediated Redox Signaling, Uncoupling Proteins, and Substrate Cycles. *Antioxidants* **2023**, *12*, 674. [CrossRef]
132. Ene, H.M.; Karry, R.; Farfara, D.; Ben-Shachar, D. Mitochondria play an essential role in the trajectory of adolescent neurodevelopment and behavior in adulthood: Evidence from a schizophrenia rat model. *Mol. Psychiatry* **2022**, *28*, 1170–1181 [CrossRef]
133. Wang, X.; Wang, W.; Li, L.; Perry, G.; Lee, H.-G.; Zhu, X. Oxidative stress and mitochondrial dysfunction in Alzheimer's disease. *Biochim. Biophys. Acta* **2014**, *1842*, 1240–1247. [CrossRef]
134. Heo, M.J.; Suh, J.H.; Lee, S.H.; Poulsen, K.L.; An, Y.A.; Moorthy, B.; Hartig, S.M.; Moore, D.D.; Kim, K.H. Aryl hydrocarbon receptor maintains hepatic mitochondrial homeostasis in mice. *Mol. Metab.* **2023**, *72*, 101717. [CrossRef] [PubMed]
135. Duarte-Hospital, C.; Tête, A.; Brial, F.; Benoit, L.; Koual, M.; Tomkiewicz, C.; Kim, M.J.; Blanc, E.B.; Coumoul, X.; Bortoli, S. Mitochondrial Dysfunction as a Hallmark of Environmental Injury. *Cells* **2021**, *11*, 110. [CrossRef] [PubMed]
136. Heath-Pagliuso, S.; Rogers, W.J.; Tullis, K.; Seidel, S.D.; Cenijn, P.H.; Brouwer, A.; Denison, M.S. Activation of the Ah receptor by tryptophan and tryptophan metabolites. *Biochemistry* **1998**, *37*, 11508–11515. [CrossRef] [PubMed]
137. Slominski, A.T.; Kim, T.-K.; Slominski, R.M.; Song, Y.; Qayyum, S.; Placha, W.; Janjetovic, Z.; Kleszczyński, K.; Atigadda, V.; Song, Y.; et al. Melatonin and Its Metabolites Can Serve as Agonists on the Aryl Hydrocarbon Receptor and Peroxisome Proliferator-Activated Receptor Gamma. *Int. J. Mol. Sci.* **2023**, *24*, 15496. [CrossRef] [PubMed]
138. Xu, C.-X.; Wang, C.; Krager, S.L.; Bottum, K.M.; Tischkau, S.A. Aryl hydrocarbon receptor activation attenuates Per1 gene induction and influences circadian clock resetting. *Toxicol. Sci.* **2013**, *132*, 368–378. [CrossRef] [PubMed]
139. Hartmann, C.; Kempf, A. Mitochondrial control of sleep. *Curr. Opin. Neurobiol.* **2023**, *81*, 102733. [CrossRef] [PubMed]
140. Wei, Y.-D.; Helleberg, H.; Rannug, U.; Rannug, A. Rapid and transient induction of CYP1A1 gene expression in human cells by the tryptophan photoproduct 6-formylindolo(3,2-b)carbazole. *Chem. Biol. Interact.* **1998**, *110*, 39–55. [CrossRef]
141. Ziv-Gal, A.; Flaws, J.A.; Mahoney, M.M.; Miller, S.R.; Zacur, H.A.; Gallicchio, L. Genetic polymorphisms in the aryl hydrocarbon receptor-signaling pathway and sleep disturbances in middle-aged women. *Sleep Med.* **2013**, *14*, 883–887. [CrossRef]
142. Frau-Méndez, M.A.; Fernández-Vega, I.; Ansoleaga, B.; Tech, R.B.; Tech, M.C.; del Rio, J.A.; Zerr, I.; Llorens, F.; Zarranz, J.J.; Ferrer, I. Fatal familial insomnia: Mitochondrial and protein synthesis machinery decline in the mediodorsal thalamus. *Brain Pathol.* **2016**, *27*, 95–106. [CrossRef]
143. Kishikawa, J.-I.; Inoue, Y.; Fujikawa, M.; Nishimura, K.; Nakanishi, A.; Tanabe, T.; Imamura, H.; Yokoyama, K. General anesthetics cause mitochondrial dysfunction and reduction of intracellular ATP levels. *PLoS ONE* **2018**, *13*, e0190213. [CrossRef]
144. Wei, H. The role of calcium dysregulation in anesthetic-mediated neurotoxicity. *Anesth. Analg.* **2011**, *113*, 972–974. [CrossRef]
145. Lee, H.-G.; Choi, S.-I.; Park, S.-K.; Park, S.-J.; Kim, N.-H.; Choi, E.-K. Alteration of glutathione metabolism and abnormal calcium accumulation in the mitochondria of hamster brain infected with scrapie agent. *Neurobiol. Aging* **2000**, *21*, 151. [CrossRef]
146. Glatzel, M.; Sepulveda-Falla, D. Losing sleep over mitochondria: A new player in the pathophysiology of fatal familial insomnia. *Brain Pathol.* **2016**, *27*, 107–108. [CrossRef] [PubMed]
147. Moon, J.-H.; Park, S.-Y. Prion peptide-mediated calcium level alteration governs neuronal cell damage through AMPK-autophagy flux. *Cell Commun. Signal.* **2020**, *18*, 109. [CrossRef] [PubMed]
148. Matteoni, S.; Matarrese, P.; Ascione, B.; Ricci-Vitiani, L.; Pallini, R.; Villani, V.; Pace, A.; Paggi, M.G.; Abbruzzese, C. Chlorpromazine induces cytotoxic autophagy in glioblastoma cells via endoplasmic reticulum stress and unfolded protein response. *J Exp. Clin. Cancer Res.* **2021**, *40*, 347. [CrossRef] [PubMed]
149. Barreca, M.L.; Iraci, N.; Biggi, S.; Cecchetti, V.; Biasini, E. Pharmacological Agents Targeting the Cellular Prion Protein. *Pathogens* **2018**, *7*, 27. [CrossRef] [PubMed]
150. Korth, C.; May, B.C.H.; Cohen, F.E.; Prusiner, S.B. Acridine and phenothiazine derivatives as pharmacotherapeutics for prion disease. *Proc. Natl. Acad. Sci. USA* **2001**, *98*, 9836–9841. [CrossRef] [PubMed]
151. Khattar, K.E.; Safi, J.; Rodriguez, A.-M.; Vignais, M.-L. Intercellular Communication in the Brain through Tunneling Nanotubes. *Cancers* **2022**, *14*, 1207. [CrossRef] [PubMed]

52. Wang, X.; Gerdes, H.-H. Transfer of mitochondria via tunneling nanotubes rescues apoptotic PC12 cells. *Cell Death Differ.* **2015**, *22*, 1181–1191. [CrossRef]
53. Savaskan, N.E.; Borchert, A.; Bräuer, A.U.; Kuhn, H. Role for glutathione peroxidase-4 in brain development and neuronal apoptosis: Specific induction of enzyme expression in reactive astrocytes following brain injury. *Free Radic. Biol. Med.* **2007**, *43*, 191–201. [CrossRef] [PubMed]
54. Mauri, S.; Favaro, M.; Bernardo, G.; Mazzotta, G.M.; Ziviani, E. Mitochondrial autophagy in the sleeping brain. *Front. Cell Dev. Biol.* **2022**, *10*, 956394. [CrossRef] [PubMed]
55. Chen, S.; Owens, G.C.; Crossin, K.L.; Edelman, D.B. Serotonin stimulates mitochondrial transport in hippocampal neurons. *Mol. Cell. Neurosci.* **2007**, *36*, 472–483. [CrossRef] [PubMed]
56. Lin, L.-C.; Nana, A.L.; Hepker, M.; Hwang, J.-H.L.; Gaus, S.E.; Spina, S.; Cosme, C.G.; Gan, L.; Grinberg, L.T.; Geschwind, D.H.; et al. Preferential tau aggregation in von Economo neurons and fork cells in frontotemporal lobar degeneration with specific MAPT variants. *Acta Neuropathol. Commun.* **2019**, *7*, 159. [CrossRef] [PubMed]
57. Kato, T. The other, forgotten genome: Mitochondrial DNA and mental disorders. *Mol. Psychiatry* **2001**, *6*, 625–633. [CrossRef] [PubMed]
58. Course, M.M.; Wang, X. Transporting mitochondria in neurons. *F1000Research* **2016**, *5*, 1735. [CrossRef]
59. Nuñez, M.T.; Chana-Cuevas, P. New Perspectives in Iron Chelation Therapy for the Treatment of Neurodegenerative Diseases. *Pharmaceuticals* **2018**, *11*, 109. [CrossRef]
60. Kupershmidt, L.; Youdim, M.B.H. The Neuroprotective Activities of the Novel Multi-Target Iron-Chelators in Models of Alzheimer's Disease, Amyotrophic Lateral Sclerosis and Aging. *Cells* **2023**, *12*, 763. [CrossRef]
61. Calderon-Montaño, J.M.; Burgos-Morón, E.; Perez-Guerrero, C.; Lopez-Lazaro, M. A Review on the Dietary Flavonoid Kaempferol. *Mini-Rev. Med. Chem.* **2011**, *11*, 298–344. [CrossRef]
62. Du, Y.-Y.; Sun, T.; Yang, Q.; Liu, Q.-Q.; Li, J.-M.; Yang, L.; Luo, L.-X. Therapeutic Potential of Kaempferol against Sleep Deprivation-Induced Cognitive Impairment: Modulation of Neuroinflammation and Synaptic Plasticity Disruption in Mice. *ACS Pharmacol. Transl. Sci.* **2023**, *6*, 1934–1944. [CrossRef]
63. Saleem, A.; Ain, Q.U.; Akhtar, M.F. Alternative Therapy of Psychosis: Potential Phytochemicals and Drug Targets in the Management of Schizophrenia. *Front. Pharmacol.* **2022**, *13*, 895668. [CrossRef]
64. Zhou, M.; Ren, H.; Han, J.; Wang, W.; Zheng, Q.; Wang, D. Protective Effects of Kaempferol against Myocardial Ischemia/Reperfusion Injury in Isolated Rat Heart via Antioxidant Activity and Inhibition of Glycogen Synthase Kinase-3β. *Oxidative Med. Cell. Longev.* **2015**, *2015*, 481405. [CrossRef] [PubMed]
65. Jope, R.S.; Roh, M.-S. Glycogen Synthase Kinase-3 (GSK3) in Psychiatric Diseases and Therapeutic Interventions. *Curr. Drug Targets* **2006**, *7*, 1421–1434. [CrossRef]
66. Mohammad, M.K.; Al-Masri, I.M.; Taha, M.O.; Al-Ghussein, M.A.; AlKhatib, H.S.; Najjar, S.; Bustanji, Y. Olanzapine inhibits glycogen synthase kinase-3beta: An investigation by docking simulation and experimental validation. *Eur. J. Pharmacol.* **2008**, *584*, 185–191. [CrossRef] [PubMed]
67. Shilovsky, G.A.; Putyatina, T.S.; Morgunova, G.V.; Seliverstov, A.V.; Ashapkin, V.V.; Sorokina, E.V.; Markov, A.V.; Skulachev, V.P. A Crosstalk between the Biorhythms and Gatekeepers of Longevity: Dual Role of Glycogen Synthase Kinase-3. *Biochemistry* **2021**, *86*, 433–448. [CrossRef] [PubMed]
68. Dozza, B.; Smith, M.A.; Perry, G.; Tabaton, M.; Strocchi, P. Regulation of glycogen synthase kinase-3beta by products of lipid peroxidation in human neuroblastoma cells. *J. Neurochem.* **2004**, *89*, 1224–1232. [CrossRef]
69. Agmon, E.; Solon, J.; Bassereau, P.; Stockwell, B.R. Modeling the effects of lipid peroxidation during ferroptosis on membrane properties. *Sci. Rep.* **2018**, *8*, 5155. [CrossRef]
70. Ohlendorf, B.; Schulz, D.; Erhard, A.; Nagel, K.; Imhoff, J.F. Geranylphenazinediol, an acetylcholinesterase inhibitor produced by a streptomyces species. *J. Nat. Prod.* **2012**, *75*, 1400–1404. [CrossRef]
71. Foster, D.J.; Bryant, Z.K.; Conn, P.J. Targeting muscarinic receptors to treat schizophrenia. *Behav. Brain Res.* **2021**, *405*, 113201. [CrossRef]
72. Wang, X.; Abbas, M.; Zhang, Y.; Elshahawi, S.I.; Ponomareva, L.V.; Cui, Z.; Van Lanen, S.G.; Sajid, I.; Voss, S.R.; Shaaban, K.A.; et al. Baraphenazines A–G, Divergent Fused Phenazine-Based Metabolites from a Himalayan Streptomyces. *J. Nat. Prod.* **2019**, *82*, 1686–1693. [CrossRef]
73. van Wezel, G.P.; McKenzie, N.L.; Nodwell, J.R. Chapter 5 Applying the genetics of secondary metabolism in model actinomycetes to the discovery of new antibiotics. In *Methods in Enzymology*, 1st ed.; Elsevier Inc.: Amsterdam, The Netherlands, 2009; Volume 458.
74. Cha, J.W.; Lee, S.I.; Kim, M.C.; Thida, M.; Lee, J.W.; Park, J.-S.; Kwon, H.C. Pontemazines A and B, phenazine derivatives containing a methylamine linkage from Streptomyces sp. UT1123 and their protective effect to HT-22 neuronal cells. *Bioorganic Med. Chem. Lett.* **2015**, *25*, 5083–5086. [CrossRef]
75. Krishnaiah, M.; Rodriguez de Almeida, N.; Udumula, V.; Song, Z.; Chhonker, Y.S.; Abdelmoaty, M.M.; Aragao do Nascimento, V.; Murry, D.J.; Conda-Sheridan, M. Synthesis, biological evaluation, and metabolic stability of phenazine derivatives as antibacterial agents. *Eur. J. Med. Chem.* **2018**, *143*, 936–947. [CrossRef] [PubMed]

176. Lavaggi, M.L.; Aguirre, G.; Boiani, L.; Orelli, L.; García, B.; Cerecetto, H.; González, M. Pyrimido[1,2-a]quinoxaline 6-oxide and phenazine 5,10-dioxide derivatives and related compounds as growth inhibitors of Trypanosoma cruzi. *Eur. J. Med. Chem.* **2008**, *43*, 1737–1741. [CrossRef] [PubMed]
177. Kato, S.; Shindo, K.; Yamagishi, Y.; Matsuoka, M.; Kawai, H.; Mochizuki, J. Phenazoviridin, a novel free radical scavenger from Streptomyces sp. taxonomy, fermentation, isolation, structure elucidation and biological properties. *J. Antibiot.* **1993**, *46*, 1485–1493. [CrossRef]
178. Laxmi, M.; Bhat, S.G. Characterization of pyocyanin with radical scavenging and antibiofilm properties isolated from Pseudomonas aeruginosa strain BTRY1. *3 Biotech* **2016**, *6*, 27. [CrossRef]
179. Alatawneh, N.; Meijler, M.M. Unraveling the Antibacterial and Iron Chelating Activity of N-Oxide Hydroxy-Phenazine natural Products and Synthetic Analogs against Staphylococcus aureus. *Isr. J. Chem.* **2023**, *63*, e202200112. [CrossRef]
180. Edinoff, A.N.; Armistead, G.; Rosa, C.A.; Anderson, A.; Patil, R.; Cornett, E.M.; Murnane, K.S.; Kaye, A.M.; Kaye, A.D. Phenothiazines and their Evolving Roles in Clinical Practice: A Narrative Review. *Health Psychol. Res.* **2022**, *10*, 38930. [CrossRef] [PubMed]
181. Heitmann, A.S.B.; Zanjani, A.A.H.; Klenow, M.B.; Mularski, A.; Sønder, S.L.; Lund, F.W.; Boye, T.L.; Dias, C.; Bendix, P.M.; Simonsen, A.C.; et al. Phenothiazines alter plasma membrane properties and sensitize cancer cells to injury by inhibiting annexin-mediated repair. *J. Biol. Chem.* **2021**, *297*, 101012. [CrossRef]
182. Boonnoy, P.; Jarerattanachat, V.; Karttunen, M.; Wong-Ekkabut, J. Bilayer Deformation, Pores, and Micellation Induced by Oxidized Lipids. *J. Phys. Chem. Lett.* **2015**, *6*, 4884–4888. [CrossRef]
183. Wu, C.-H.; Bai, L.-Y.; Tsai, M.-H.; Chu, P.-C.; Chiu, C.-F.; Chen, M.Y.; Chiu, S.-J.; Chiang, J.-H.; Weng, J.-R. Pharmacological exploitation of the phenothiazine antipsychotics to develop novel antitumor agents–A drug repurposing strategy. *Sci. Rep.* **2016**, *6*, 27540. [CrossRef]
184. Voronova, O.; Zhuravkov, S.; Korotkova, E.; Artamonov, A.; Plotnikov, E. Antioxidant Properties of New Phenothiazine Derivatives. *Antioxidants* **2022**, *11*, 1371. [CrossRef]
185. Keynes, R.G.; Karchevskaya, A.; Riddall, D.; Griffiths, C.H.; Bellamy, T.C.; Chan, A.W.E.; Selwood, D.L.; Garthwaite, J. N10 carbonyl-substituted phenothiazines inhibiting lipid peroxidation and associated nitric oxide consumption powerfully protect brain tissue against oxidative stress. *Chem. Biol. Drug Des.* **2019**, *94*, 1680–1693. [CrossRef]
186. Iuga, C.; Campero, A.; Vivier-Bunge, A. Antioxidant vs. prooxidant action of phenothiazine in a biological environment in the presence of hydroxyl and hydroperoxyl radicals: A quantum chemistry study. *RSC Adv.* **2015**, *5*, 14678–14689. [CrossRef]
187. Yue, Y.; Kong, L.; Wang, J.; Li, C.; Tan, L.; Su, H.; Xu, Y. Regional Abnormality of Grey Matter in Schizophrenia: Effect from the Illness or Treatment? *PLoS ONE* **2016**, *11*, e0147204. [CrossRef]
188. Martínez, A.; Ibarra, I.A.; Vargas, R. A quantum chemical approach representing a new perspective concerning agonist and antagonist drugs in the context of schizophrenia and Parkinson's disease. *PLoS ONE* **2019**, *14*, e0224691. [CrossRef]
189. Goode-Romero, G.; Dominguez, L.; Martínez, A. Electron Donor–Acceptor Properties of Different Muscarinic Ligands: On the Road to Control Schizophrenia. *J. Chem. Inf. Model.* **2021**, *61*, 5117–5124. [CrossRef] [PubMed]
190. Ho, B.C.; Andreasen, N.C.; Ziebell, S.; Pierson, R.; Magnotta, V. Long-term antipsychotic treatment and brain volumes: A longitudinal study of first-episode schizophrenia. *Arch. Gen. Psychiatry* **2011**, *68*, 128–137. [CrossRef]
191. Engwa, G.A.; Ayuk, E.L.; Igbojekwe, B.U.; Unaegbu, M. Potential Antioxidant Activity of New Tetracyclic and Pentacyclic Nonlinear Phenothiazine Derivatives. *Biochem. Res. Int.* **2016**, *2016*, 9896575. [CrossRef] [PubMed]
192. Liang, Z.; Currais, A.; Soriano-Castell, D.; Schubert, D.; Maher, P. Natural products targeting mitochondria: Emerging therapeutics for age-associated neurological disorders. *Pharmacol. Ther.* **2021**, *221*, 107749. [CrossRef] [PubMed]
193. Imran, M.; Ghorat, F.; Ul-Haq, I.; Ur-Rehman, H.; Aslam, F.; Heydari, M.; Shariati, M.A.; Okuskhanova, E.; Yessimbekov, Z.; Thiruvengadam, M.; et al. Lycopene as a Natural Antioxidant Used to Prevent Human Health Disorders. *Antioxidants* **2020**, *9*, 706. [CrossRef] [PubMed]
194. Urquiaga, I.; Leighton, F. Plant polyphenol antioxidants and oxidative stress. *Biol. Res.* **2000**, *33*, 55–64. [CrossRef] [PubMed]
195. Kumar, N.; Goel, N. Phenolic acids: Natural versatile molecules with promising therapeutic applications. *Biotechnol. Rep.* **2019**, *24*, e00370. [CrossRef] [PubMed]
196. Jakubczyk, K.; Drużga, A.; Katarzyna, J.; Skonieczna-Żydecka, K. Antioxidant Potential of Curcumin—A Meta-Analysis of Randomized Clinical Trials. *Antioxidants* **2020**, *9*, 1092. [CrossRef] [PubMed]
197. Nagle, D.G.; Ferreira, D.; Zhou, Y.-D. Epigallocatechin-3-gallate (EGCG): Chemical and biomedical perspectives. *Phytochemistry* **2006**, *67*, 1849–1855. [CrossRef] [PubMed]
198. Li, Z.; Geng, Y.-N.; Jiang, J.-D.; Kong, W.-J. Antioxidant and anti-inflammatory activities of berberine in the treatment of diabetes mellitus. *Evid. Based Complement. Altern. Med.* **2014**, *2014*, 289264. [CrossRef]
199. Deepika; Maurya, P.K. Health Benefits of Quercetin in Age-Related Diseases. *Molecules* **2022**, *27*, 2498. [CrossRef] [PubMed]
200. Chen, A.Y.; Chen, Y.C. A review of the dietary flavonoid, kaempferol on human health and cancer chemoprevention. *Food Chem.* **2013**, *138*, 2099–2107. [CrossRef]
201. Frankel, E.N. The antioxidant and nutritional effects of tocopherols, ascorbic acid and beta-carotene in relation to processing of edible oils. *Bibl. Nutr. Dieta* **1989**, *43*, 297–312. [CrossRef]
202. Liu, D.; Gao, Y.; Liu, J.; Huang, Y.; Yin, J.; Feng, Y.; Shi, L.; Meloni, B.P.; Zhang, C.; Zheng, M.; et al. Intercellular mitochondrial transfer as a means of tissue revitalization. *Signal Transduct. Target. Ther.* **2021**, *6*, 65. [CrossRef]

203. Katrangi, E.; D'Souza, G.; Boddapati, S.V.; Kulawiec, M.; Singh, K.K.; Bigger, B.; Weissig, V. Xenogenic transfer of isolated murine mitochondria into human rho0 cells can improve respiratory function. *Rejuvenation Res.* **2007**, *10*, 561–570. [CrossRef]
204. Pacak, C.A.; Preble, J.M.; Kondo, H.; Seibel, P.; Levitsky, S.; del Nido, P.J.; Cowan, D.B.; McCully, J.D. Actin-dependent mitochondrial internalization in cardiomyocytes: Evidence for rescue of mitochondrial function. *Biol. Open* **2015**, *4*, 622–626. [CrossRef] [PubMed]
205. Berridge, M.V.; Schneider, R.T.; McConnell, M.J. Mitochondrial Transfer from Astrocytes to Neurons following Ischemic Insult: Guilt by Association? *Cell Metab.* **2016**, *24*, 376–378. [CrossRef] [PubMed]
206. Pour, P.A.; Hosseinian, S.; Kheradvar, A. Mitochondrial transplantation in cardiomyocytes: Foundation, methods, and outcomes. *Am. J. Physiol. Cell Physiol.* **2021**, *321*, C489–C503. [CrossRef] [PubMed]
207. Cowan, D.B.; Yao, R.; Thedsanamoorthy, J.K.; Zurakowski, D.; del Nido, P.J.; McCully, J.D. Transit and fusion of exogenous mitochondria in human heart cells. *Nat. Sci. Rep.* **2017**, *7*, 17450. [CrossRef]
208. Zhang, T.-G.; Miao, C.-Y. Mitochondrial transplantation as a promising therapy for mitochondrial diseases. *Acta Pharm. Sin. B* **2023**, *13*, 1028–1035. [CrossRef]
209. Scheiblich, H.; Dansokho, C.; Mercan, D.; Schmidt, S.V.; Bousset, L.; Wischhof, L.; Eikens, F.; Odainic, A.; Spitzer, J.; Griep, A.; et al. Microglia jointly degrade fibrillar alpha-synuclein cargo by distribution through tunneling nanotubes. *Cell* **2021**, *184*, 5089–5106.e21. [CrossRef]
210. Geng, Z.; Guan, S.; Wang, S.; Yu, Z.; Liu, T.; Du, S.; Zhu, C. Intercellular mitochondrial transfer in the brain, a new perspective for targeted treatment of central nervous system diseases. *CNS Neurosci. Ther.* **2023**, *29*, 3121–3135. [CrossRef]
211. Ren, D.; Zheng, P.; Zou, S.; Gong, Y.; Wang, Y.; Duan, J.; Deng, J.; Chen, H.; Feng, J.; Zhong, C.; et al. GJA1-20K Enhances Mitochondria Transfer from Astrocytes to Neurons via Cx43-TnTs After Traumatic Brain Injury. *Cell. Mol. Neurobiol.* **2021**, *42*, 1887–1895. [CrossRef]

Disclaimer/Publisher's Note: The statements, opinions and data contained in all publications are solely those of the individual author(s) and contributor(s) and not of MDPI and/or the editor(s). MDPI and/or the editor(s) disclaim responsibility for any injury to people or property resulting from any ideas, methods, instructions or products referred to in the content.

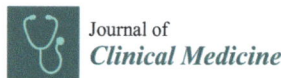

Review

The Cyclical Battle of Insomnia and Mental Health Impairment in Firefighters: A Narrative Review

Angelia M. Holland-Winkler *, Daniel R. Greene and Tiffany J. Oberther

Department of Kinesiology, Augusta University, 3109 Wrightsboro Road, Augusta, GA 30909, USA; dagreene@augusta.edu (D.R.G.); toberther@augusta.edu (T.J.O.)
* Correspondence: awinkler@augusta.edu

Abstract: The occupational requirements of full-time non-administrative firefighters include shift-work schedules and chronic exposure to alerting emergency alarms, hazardous working conditions, and psychologically traumatic events that they must attend and respond to. These compiling and enduring aspects of the career increase the firefighter's risk for insomnia and mental health conditions compared to the general population. Poor sleep quality and mental health impairments are known to coincide with and contribute to the symptom severity of one another. Thus, it is important to determine approaches that may improve sleep and/or mental health specifically for firefighters, as their occupation varies in many aspects from any other occupation. This review will discuss symptoms of insomnia and mental health conditions such as PTSD, anxiety, depression, substance abuse, and suicide in firefighters. The influencing factors of sleep and mental health will be examined including anxiety sensitivity, emotional regulation, and distress tolerance. Current sleep and mental health interventions specific to full-time firefighters are limited in number; however, the existing experimental studies will be outlined. Lastly, this review will provide support for exploring exercise as a possible intervention that may benefit the sleep and mental health of this population.

Keywords: sleep quality; first responders; PTSD; anxiety; depression; emotional regulation; substance abuse; suicide

1. Introduction

The occupational demands of firefighters are often stressful, tense, and volatile [1]. They must be prepared to respond to a wide range of unpredictable and often hazardous emergencies. Although firefighters are thoroughly trained to be safe in dangerous situations, they are still highly susceptible to injury. They also face psychological trauma as they are the first to respond to suffering individuals (i.e., a child in trouble or suffering) [2–4]. At the fire station, they are exposed to loud shrilling emergency alerting alarms, during both the day and night, which frequently and rapidly activate their sympathetic nervous system [5,6]. These physical and psychological stressors encountered every working shift have been shown to lead to increased risk for major health conditions such as cardiovascular disease, cancer, and depression [7–9].

In addition to these stressors, most firefighters are shift-workers. Shift schedules vary across fire departments; fire departments may adopt a 24 h on/48 h off or 48 h on/96 h off schedule, while others may adopt a more complex schedule like the Kelly schedule which consists of 24 h on/24 h off/24 h on/24 h off/24 h on/96 h off [10,11]. Some firefighters may even work shifts that last as long as 72 h [12]. During working shifts, firefighters are expected to be on call and respond immediately to emergency alarms [5]. This required alertness significantly impacts sleep while on shift and may also impact sleep patterns off shift as well, leading to sleep deprivations, severe circadian dysrhythmias, and possibly chronically impaired sleep patterns [7,13]. The internal circadian rhythm synchronizes with external environmental cues including light, physical activity, and melatonin secretion with light exposure being the most dominant regulator [14]. The misalignment of the circadian rhythm with the 24 h outside environment may lead to a circadian rhythm disorder which negatively affects sleep and may lead to health conditions including metabolic, cognitive, cardiovascular, and gastrointestinal impairments [15].

Sleep is vitally important to both physical and mental health [16]. Sleep recommendations include seven to nine hours of sleep for adults, with continuous cycles of rapid eye movement (REM) and nonrapid eye movement (NREM) sleep over the course of the total sleep period [17]. Each cycle of REM and NREM occurs every 90–120 min, with it taking at least one hour to reach NREM sleep [18]. REM sleep occurs after slow-wave sleep and allows for emotional memory processing, while NREM sleep is required for optimal wakefulness and cognitive function the following day [19–23]. Seven to nine hours of sleep is recommended to allow for three to six REM/NREM cycles per night [24]. This consistency of sufficient sleep patterns helps regulate circadian rhythm which in turn promotes sufficient sleep patterns and health.

Optimal wakefulness and cognitive function occurring from NREM sleep are required for the intense physical and mental obligations of firefighting [25]. In addition, emotional memory processing and thought processing that occurs through REM sleep is valuable to the long-term psychological and even physical health of firefighters [26–28]. However, firefighters commonly suffer from both insomnia and mental health conditions due to the nature of their occupation. Mental health conditions common in firefighters include post-traumatic stress disorder (PTSD), depression, anxiety, and substance abuse which may cause a greater risk for suicidal thoughts and attempts [7,29–31]. Many studies have sought to determine the relationship between insomnia and mental health as well as interventions that may improve these conditions in firefighters [10,30]. This narrative review will discuss the prevalence, mechanisms, and relationship of insomnia and mental health disorders in firefighters as well as interventions that have been utilized to improve these conditions.

2. Insomnia and Firefighters

2.1. Insomnia Evaluation

In general, insomnia occurs when someone has difficulty sleeping [32]. Diagnosed clinical insomnia can be categorized as acute insomnia and/or chronic insomnia. Acute insomnia occurs when a person has difficulty going to sleep and/or staying asleep at least three days per week for a period of one week to three months [33]. There are multiple types of acute insomnia such as transient and sub-chronic insomnia, but for the scope of this review, these sub-categories of acute insomnia will not be discussed in detail [33]. A diagnosis of chronic insomnia may occur if a person has difficulty going to and/or staying asleep at least three days per week for at least three months, despite having sufficient time to sleep. Additional criteria for chronic insomnia include significant daytime impairment or distress [33–35].

Schutte-Rodin et al. [36] describe the guidelines for a clinical evaluation of insomnia which include a thorough sleep history and a detailed medical, substance, and psychiatric history. It is recommended for the evaluation to consist of the following subjective reports or measures: medical and psychiatric questionnaire, subjective sleep assessment (i.e., Epworth Sleepiness Scale), and a two-week sleep log. Polysomnography and actigraphy are additional objective assessments that may provide beneficial data for further insomnia evaluation [36].

Population-based epidemiological studies over the past few decades have reported variable rates of insomnia in general populations, but the consensus from those studies is that 30–36% of adults report having at least one nighttime sleep-related symptom of insomnia, while 10–15% of the population has at least one nighttime sleep-related and one daytime fatigue-related symptom of insomnia [26,37]. However, when more rigorous insomnia criteria are used to determine insomnia rates (i.e., diagnostic criteria from the Diagnostic and Statistical Manual of Mental Disorders IV; DSM IV), the prevalence in adults decreases to 6–10% [38,39]. It is therefore difficult to compare insomnia rates in various populations when different criteria are utilized.

2.2. Sleep Measures in Firefighter Studies

The terms sleep deprivation, sleep disorder, disturbed sleep patterns, clinical insomnia, and poor sleep quality are commonly used in firefighter-based sleep studies. Sleep patterns in firefighters are often assessed with the Pittsburgh Sleep Quality Index (PSQI), a validated subjective questionnaire that measures sleep quality and disturbances over a one-month period. It includes 19 items to then provide scores for seven components of sleep quality on a "0" ("best sleep quality")-to-"3" ("worst sleep quality") scale; those seven components include subjective sleep quality, sleep latency, sleep duration, habitual sleep efficiency, sleep disturbances, the use of sleep medication, and daytime dysfunction [40]. The seven scores are summed, and a score of 5 or less indicates good sleep quality, and a score of greater than 5 indicates poor sleep quality.

Another subjective sleep quality questionnaire frequently used in this population is the Epworth Sleepiness Scale (ESS) which differs from the PSQI as it assesses the likelihood of falling asleep in various daytime scenarios. The ESS asks participants to indicate, on a 4-point Likert scale, how likely they would be to fall asleep with "0" indicating "no chance of dozing" and "3" indicating a "high chance of dozing". A total score of 0–9 indicates that "you are not abnormally sleepy", a score of 10–15 indicates that "you may be excessively sleepy depending on the situation and you may want to consider seeking medical attention", and a score of 16–24 indicates that "you are excessively sleepy and should consider seeking medical attention". When compared to other clinical measures of sleep quality, it was found valid and reliable [41]. Many studies use both the PSQI and ESS to assess nocturnal sleep difficulties and daytime sleepiness together.

Lastly, the insomnia severity index (ISI) is another validated subjective questionnaire used in this population to measure insomnia severity [42]. The ISI consists of seven sleep-related questions rated on a five-point Likert scale with "0" corresponding to "no problem" and "4" corresponding to a "very severe problem". A score of 15 or higher indicates clinical insomnia with a score of 15–21 being categorized as "moderate insomnia" and 22–28 being categorized as "severe insomnia". Multiple studies have utilized objective sleep assessments such as an actigraphy motion logger which may be worn for periods of days to weeks to detect sleep patterns.

2.3. Poor Sleep Prevalence in Firefighters

The prevalence of poor sleep quality in firefighters has been reported by various studies and differs based on country and sleep quality measures. In a large study by Horn et al. [30], 880 current and retired United States firefighters completed a web-based ISI and 52.7% reported clinically significant insomnia symptoms with 19.2% reporting nightmare problems. Cary et al. [7] showed that 59% of full-time firefighters in a metropolitan area of the United States reported sleep deprivation which was measured with the PSQI and ESS questionnaires as well as a 3-day actigraphy motion logger. They considered the firefighter to have a disturbed sleep pattern if they had at least two of the following sleep issues: sleep duration <6 h, sleep efficiency <85%, sleep latency >30 min, or wake after sleep onset >30 min. Billings et al. [11] assessed sleep quality in 109 full-time shift-working firefighters in the United States using the PSQI and found that 73% reported poor sleep quality; those that worked a second job had significantly poorer sleep quality than those who did not. Thus, in the United States, the prevalence of poor sleep quality in firefighters ranges from 52 to 73% in studies that include over 100 participants.

Sleep quality has been assessed in firefighters outside of the United States with similar results. Mehrdad et al. [43] assessed sleep quality in 427 Iranian firefighters using the Persian version of the PSQI. They received an 88.7% response rate with 69.9% reporting poor sleep quality. Lim et al. [44] assessed the sleep quality of 657 full-time firefighters in a metropolitan area of South Korea using the PSQI. In total, 48.7% reported poor sleep quality; however, shift-workers reported significantly higher levels of poor sleep quality (51.6%) than the non-shift-workers (38.5%). In a large study by Cramm et al. [10], 69% of 1217 volunteer and full-time Canadian firefighters self-reported their sleep quality as "fair" to "very poor", and 21.3% were found to have clinical insomnia based on the ISI scores. Thus, the prevalence of poor sleep quality ranges depending on the assessment and the working schedule of the firefighters but is typically higher than the general population of the area [10,11,26,45].

The incidence of chronic insomnia in firefighters is difficult to accurately determine based on the results from most experimental or observational sleep studies in this population as the sleep assessments are typically based on a one-month period, whereas a diagnosis of chronic insomnia requires a minimum of a three-month assessment or report of sleep difficulty. However, since firefighters are more likely to have sleep impairments than the general population, it can be assumed that the nature of their occupation may be the overarching factor resulting in the poor sleep quality found with the one-month assessments. Thus, if the firefighter has a history of employment longer than three months, it could be assumed that the one-month assessment of poor sleep quality would occur throughout employment and be considered chronic. However, this is an assumption and needs further exploration.

3. Mental Health and Firefighters

Firefighters are regularly exposed to significant physical, emotional, and psychological challenges. As part of their daily routine, every call exposes them to a potentially traumatic event. As such, it comes with little surprise that firefighters often report elevated prevalence rates associated with mental health disorders. A recent systematic review examining the mental health of firefighters relative to the general population has concluded firefighters are significantly more likely to experience PTSD, depression, and anxiety [46]. Wolffe et al. [31] assessed the overall prevalence of mental health disorders among UK firefighters relative to the general English population. Approximately 12% of firefighters reported anxiety, 10% reported depression, and 5% reported PTSD. In contrast, approximately 6% of the general UK population reported anxiety, 3% reported depression, and just under 5% reported PTSD [31].

3.1. Anxiety

According to the Diagnostic and Statistical Manual of Mental Disorder (DSM-5), anxiety is a normal response to stress, while an anxiety disorder is associated with intense feelings of excessive worry and apprehension. Additionally, the DSM-5 describes an anxiety disorder as a chronic condition in which individuals experience symptoms on most days (i.e., more days than not) over the previous 6 months [47]. While anxiety is inherently a negative stress response, not all stress negatively impacts you. There are two distinct responses individuals experience in the presence of stress. Individuals can feel motivated, excited, and approach a stressful situation as a challenge to overcome. This is referred to as eustress or positive stress and can be beneficial for overall health and wellness [48]. However, stress can promote feelings of anxiety, discomfort, and decrease motivation. This type of stress is negative and referred to as distress [48]. While there are specific stressors that typically promote eustress (e.g., exercise/physical activity) or distress (e.g., traumatic events) there are individual characteristics that act to protect one from significant distress such as anxiety sensitivity and emotional regulation [49]. As firefighters are naturally exposed to potentially traumatic events, these individual characteristics could be a significant factor concerning mental health in this population.

As mentioned above, firefighters are exposed to extremely stressful situations and often experience increased anxiety relative to the general population. To highlight this, a recent report identified a career as a firefighter to be the second most stressful job in the United States [50]. Wolffe et al. [31] reported that firefighters are more than twice as likely to experience anxiety relative to the general population. The Health Hazard Evaluation

Program reported that 53% of firefighters experienced symptoms of Generalized Anxiety Disorder (GAD) [51]. A recent meta-analysis assessed 8096 first responders and reported 60% met criteria for mild anxiety, 27% met criteria for moderate anxiety, and 14% met criteria for severe anxiety [52]. While the symptoms of anxiety can be severe and debilitating on their own, individuals living with higher levels of anxiety are more susceptible to other mental health conditions. It has been well established that firefighters experience significant occupational stress, and reports indicate that occupational stress is a significant predictor of PTSD symptomology in firefighters [53]. Occupational stress in firefighters has been linked to numerous other mental health concerns. First, as mentioned above, individuals can have a more positive (i.e., eustress) or more negative (i.e., distress) response to external stressors. While occupational stress is inherently negative, increased occupational stress in firefighters has been correlated to increased PTSD symptom severity, depression, and anxiety [54,55]. Firefighters with higher occupational stress are more likely to experience severe mental health disorders, and this relationship is further exacerbated by disturbances in sleep.

According to the UK Firefighter Contamination Survey, 46% of firefighters self-reported their mental health to be a significant factor impacting their sleep disturbance [31]. Yook et al. [56] examined the relationship between occupational stress and sleep quality in 705 male firefighters. The firefighters were evenly divided into a low stress, medium stress, or high stress tertile group. Firefighters in the high stress group experienced significantly worse outcomes in subjective sleep quality, sleep latency, sleep duration, habitual sleep efficiency, sleep disturbances, the use of sleeping medication, and daytime dysfunction relative to both low and medium stress groups. Further, firefighters in the medium stress group reported significantly worse outcomes in subjective sleep quality, sleep disturbances, and daytime dysfunction relative to the low stress group [56]. While the prevalence of anxiety has been linked to disturbed sleep, this is a reciprocal relationship. Data from the National Canadian Mental Health Survey indicated firefighters with insomnia to be 7.15 times more likely to suffer from GAD relative to firefighters without insomnia [10]. Simply by examining anxiety, the cyclical relationship between mental health conditions and insomnia can be seen in firefighters.

3.2. Depression

Another leading mental health concern for firefighters is depression. According to DSM-5 criteria, an individual must experience five or more major depressive disorder (MDD) symptoms during the same two-week period to be diagnosed with MDD. These symptoms include a depressed mood, a diminished interest in activities that used to be pleasurable, a significant change in body weight without apparent effort, insomnia, significant fatigue, feelings of worthlessness, decreased concentration, suicidal ideation, and psychomotor agitation [47]. While estimates vary, it is generally accepted that firefighters experience elevated depression and MDD relative to the general population. A large study estimates the 12-month depression prevalence to be between 5.5 and 6.0% in the general population [57] where estimates are significantly higher in firefighter populations (e.g., 40% [30]). Within the firefighter population, there are significant risk factors associated with experiencing greater levels of depression. Rescue and disaster workers who were exposed to a disaster were significantly more likely to experience depression at 7 and 13 months following the event relative to rescue and disaster workers who were not exposed to a similar event [58]. Specifically, 21.7% of the exposed workers experienced depression, while 12.6% of non-exposed workers experienced similar feelings of depression 13 months after the event [58].

While it is clear that firefighters are more likely to experience elevated depression and MDD relative to the general population, it is equally important to explore specific comorbidities linked to depression within this population. Individuals living with MDD have reported a significant increase in other mental health disorders including anxiety [59], alcohol and drug use [60], and suicidal ideation/attempts [61]. These relationships are present and often exacerbated in firefighters. In a sample of 169 firefighters exposed to a traumatic event, 53.3% reported depression and 57% met the full DSM-IV criteria for PTSD. Further, depression and PTSD were significantly correlated [62]. In addition to other mental health disorders, depression has been linked to other psychological disturbances.

There is a strong amount of evidence linking insomnia as a risk factor for depression [26]. Even non-depressed individuals have a twofold risk for developing depression if they have insomnia compared to people that do not suffer from sleep difficulties [63]. Firefighters suffering from disturbed sleep were shown to be twice as likely to have anxiety or depression. Further, firefighters with sleeping problems were over four times as likely to experience a mental health concern [31]. Cramm et al. [10] assessed 1217 firefighters from the National Canadian Mental Health Survey and reported firefighters with insomnia to be 7.91 times more likely to experience MDD than firefighters without insomnia. Similarly, Horn et al. [30] assessed 880 United States firefighters with cross-sectional surveys and found that 39.6% had clinically significant symptoms of depression, 52.7% had insomnia symptoms, and 19.2% had nightmares; they suggested that insomnia may increase the risk for depression through the impairment of emotional regulation (described below).

3.3. PTSD

According to the DSM-5 criteria, an individual is likely to have PTSD following exposure to a traumatic event if they exhibit symptoms of re-experiencing, avoidance, negative alterations in cognitions and mood, and hyperarousal [47]. Firefighters are at a significantly higher risk of experiencing PTSD symptoms. Specific studies have estimated the rate of PTSD symptoms to affect approximately 17% of Canadian firefighters [29], 18% of German firefighters [64], and 22% of American firefighters [29]. In a sample of 3289 firefighters, 13% (i.e., 432) reported symptoms of PTSD [65], and a recent review reported the PTSD prevalence in firefighters to be as high as 57% [66]. This is striking as estimates of the PTSD prevalence in civilian populations have been estimated as low as 2.3–2.9% [67]. Firefighters with PTSD symptoms were significantly more likely to suffer from work-related injuries, chronic musculoskeletal disorders, burnout, and poor physical condition [65]. Further, Fullerton et al. [58] examined disaster workers who were exposed to a traumatic event relative to comparison workers who were not exposed. Their results indicate that 16.7% of exposed workers reported PTSD while only 1.9% of non-exposed workers reported PTSD 13 months following the incident.

PTSD is a trauma- and stress-related disorder, but prior to 2013, PTSD was classified as an anxiety disorder [47]. Thus, PTSD shares numerous risk factors and comorbidities with other mental health conditions. According to data from the National Comorbidity Survey, of those diagnosed with PTSD, 54% reported having a major depressive episode, 28% reported having GAD, 28% reported alcohol abuse/dependence, and over 43% identified as having three or more other diagnosed conditions [68]. Specifically in firefighters, PTSD symptom severity has been associated with numerous other mental health concerns. Bing-Canar et al. [69] assessed 632 trauma-exposed firefighters and found PTSD symptoms to significantly predict suicide risk. A recent systematic review has identified anxiety, depression, work-related injuries, and chronic musculoskeletal disorders as significant comorbidities that predict PTSD prevalence among firefighters [70].

Insomnia and other sleep disturbances are diagnostic symptoms of PTSD and not easily treated. Sleep disturbances mediate PTSD, leaving suffering individuals to function poorly during the day in addition to promoting poorer PTSD-related clinical outcomes such as increased alcohol use, poorer physical and mental health, and reduced overall quality of life [28]. With sleep disturbances being resistant to first-line treatments for PTSD (i.e., pharmacotherapy [71] and cognitive behavioral therapy [72]), firefighters suffering from PTSD and insomnia may need multiple forms of treatment; however, this needs further exploration.

3.4. Obsessive–Compulsive Disorder (OCD)

While the prevalence of OCD is not as widespread as other mental health concerns, firefighters are at an increased risk for living with OCD. According to a large survey of 10,649 firefighters, 1.6% reported having OCD [31]. Despite the relatively low prevalence of OCD in firefighters, it is important to reference the general population. A large epidemiological study of 25,180 individuals from Iran found the prevalence of OCD to be 1.8%, with females significantly more likely to experience OCD relative to males [73]. Further, a recent meta-analysis highlights the notion that women are 1.6 times more likely to experience OCD relative to men [74]. Given the relatively similar prevalence rates of OCD in firefighters and the general population, the sex differences highlight an interesting notion. Specifically, over 95% of all US firefighters between 2011 and 2015 were male [75]. Therefore, it is reasonable to conclude that the 1.6% prevalence rate of OCD in predominantly male firefighters is significantly greater than the average OCD rate reported by men. Specifically, the prevalence of OCD has been estimated at 0.7% and 2.8% for males and females, respectively [73].

OCD has been linked to numerous other mental health concerns. Hofer et al. found strong evidence linking prior OCD to an increased risk of GAD and social phobias [76]. Individuals living with OCD have a significantly greater risk of suicidal thoughts and actions. The presence of depression further exacerbates the increased risk of suicidal ideations [77]. Specifically in firefighters, there is evidence that the demands of the job can lead to an increased risk in developing OCD or OCD symptoms [78].

3.5. Suicide

Suicide is another mental health concern that is of paramount importance with respect to firefighters. Overall, first responders have been identified as a population at increased risk for numerous mental health concerns including suicide [79]. Within the general population, 13.5% have reported suicidal thoughts, 3.9% have reported suicidal plans, and 4.6% have reported a suicide attempt [80]. While these numbers are striking, firefighters have reported significantly greater suicide behaviors. Specifically, 46.8% of firefighters have reported suicidal thoughts, 19.2% have reported making a suicide plan, and 15.5% have experienced a suicidal action [81]. Suicide takes the lives of 800,000 people each year [82]. While it is important to highlight the increased risk firefighters face with respect to suicidal thoughts and actions, it is equally important to understand other risk factors associated with suicide.

Suicide has been associated with numerous other mental health outcomes. Survey results indicate both PTSD and GAD to be significant predictors for suicidal ideation and attempts [83] in a large sample of adults from the general population. This relationship has also been shown in firefighters. Firefighters with greater PTSD symptom severity [84] and levels of depression [85] reported a significantly greater risk of suicide. Suicidal ideation and attempts have also been linked to other psychological factors such as sleep. A National Comorbidity Survey was filled out by 8098 adults in the United States and assessed to determine the association between sleep, mental disorders, suicidal ideation, and suicide attempts over the past 12 months and lifetime. The results demonstrated that short sleep increases the chances of suicidal ideation and suicide attempts, regardless of mental conditions. Furthermore, suicidal ideation and short sleep was shown to increase the odds of a suicide attempt and was additionally related to the presence of substance use disorders [86]. Vargos de Barros et al. [16] assessed six mental health conditions in 303 Brazilian firefighters which included stress, depression, anxiety, suicidal ideation, alcohol use disorders, and general health with subscales of a desire for death, psychosomatic problems, and sleep disturbances. Of the 303 firefighters, 51% had sleep disturbances which were significantly related to the presence of psychological distress and psychosomatic alterations. Suicidal ideation was found in 15% of the firefighters and unhealthy alcohol use in 31%; both conditions trended toward a significant association with sleep disturbances ($p < 0.085$). A case study described an older man with poor sleep quality, excessive daytime sleepiness, a depressed mood, and suicidal ideation with active suicide plans that was treated for sleep apnea without antidepressant medication [87]. He responded well to the sleep apnea treatment (nCAP) and his suicidal ideation and depression resolved, which demonstrates the need to treat sleep conditions to improve the outcomes of other likely associated mental conditions.

3.6. Substance Abuse

Firefighters have been identified as a population at significantly greater risk for substance abuse. A recent national survey of 674 firefighters concluded over 48% displayed heavy drinking behaviors and over 43% met the criteria for binge drinking [88]. Relative to the general population, these numbers are significantly elevated. According to a recent meta-analysis including six national surveys, about 25% of the United States' adult population reported binge drinking behavior [89]. Interestingly, recent reports indicate the general female population displays significantly lower levels of binge drinking behavior (i.e., about 13.5% [90]). Thus, Haddock et al. [90] assessed drinking behavior in a large sample of female firefighters (N = 1913). Their results indicate about 40% of female firefighters reported binge drinking. Even though female firefighters only account for roughly 5% of the firefighter population, they also experience a significant increase in substance abuse behavior [91].

Firefighters are also at an increased risk for using other psychoactive substances. In a sample of 112 firefighters, 58% displayed binge drinking behavior, 20% identified as nicotine users, and 5% met criteria for caffeine overuse (i.e., >700 mg/day) [7]. While less is known about specific drug use among firefighters, there is some evidence of anxiolytic drug use. Specifically, in a recent survey of 711 military firefighters, the anxiolytic drug use was 9.9% [92]. Another survey on firefighters and psychoactive substance use included questionnaires on tobacco, alcohol, prescribed medication, and illicit drug use. Among the 168 male firefighters included, 89.9% reported alcohol consumption, 38.1% reported smoking tobacco, 2.4% reported taking prescribed medications, and 1.2% reported illicit drug use [93]. While it is possible firefighters are not accurately self-reporting medication and drug use, the main area of concern among this population appears to be alcohol use. While substance abuse is a very important mental health concern, it has also been linked to other mental health conditions such as PTSD [94], depression [7], and sleep quality [7] in firefighters. As mentioned above, firefighters can be under extreme occupational stress and might seek external coping mechanisms. Alcohol consumption has been identified as one of the most prominent coping strategies used by firefighters in response to occupational stress [95,96]. Further, alcohol consumption has been associated with suicide risk among firefighters [69]. To explore this phenomenon, Martin et al. [97] examined the impact of alcohol dependence on suicide risk in 2883 male firefighters. Their results indicated a significant association between alcohol dependance and suicide risk in firefighters. Additionally, they found evidence linking alcohol dependance to increases in depression, which further predicted suicide risk factors [97]. This highlights the cyclical nature of mental health disorders among firefighters.

Alcohol is a substance that causes sleepiness and may help non-alcoholic healthy individuals fall asleep faster and have better NREM sleep; however, it may disrupt sleep during the second half of the night. Both periods of binge drinking and alcohol abstinence have been shown to disrupt sleep [98]. Smith et al. [99] assessed sleep, mental health, and alcohol use in 639 urban career firefighters and found a significant positive correlation between sleep disturbance severity and alcohol use severity as well as alcohol use for coping reasons. In addition, there was a significant positive correlation between PTSD severity and alcohol use severity and alcohol use for coping reasons which was even stronger when sleep disturbances were high in the firefighters. The cyclical nature of these impairments underlines the importance of finding treatment options that may improve the health of more than one condition.

3.7. Implications

Based on the evidence above, mental health conditions such as anxiety, depression, PTSD, substance abuse, and suicide risk factors are often comorbidities of each other and with sleep disturbance. However, it is important to note that one is not caused by the other. That is, while individuals living with MDD are more likely to be diagnosed with GAD, both MDD and GAD have significant and independent impacts on mental health [100]. Further, Elhai et al. assessed the overlapping symptoms associated with PTSD, anxiety, and other mood disorders. After controlling for overlapping symptoms, the overall PTSD prevalence only decreased by 0.39%, from 6.81 to 6.42% [68]. This suggests that symptoms from a specific mental health condition will not cause another mental health condition but rather increase the susceptibility to separate, independent comorbidities. Taken together, this highlights the cyclical battle firefighters face with mental health and insomnia.

4. Factors Influencing Sleep and Mental Health

4.1. Anxiety Sensitivity

While firefighters are exposed to traumatic events that increase their risk of experiencing negative mental health outcomes, there may be specific traits that protect against this. One individual trait that may influence mental health outcomes following exposure to a traumatic event is an individual's fear of arousal-related situations (i.e., anxiety sensitivity). According to Taylor et al. [101], anxiety sensitivity can be accessed via the 18-item, self-report anxiety sensitivity index (ASI-3). The ASI-3 is a valid assessment of general (i.e., global) anxiety sensitivity and physical (i.e., fear induced by increased heart rate), cognitive (i.e., fear induced by concentration difficulties), and social (i.e., fear induced by being observed in anxiety-producing situations) concerns [101]. General anxiety sensitivity has been shown to significantly affect the symptoms of PTSD, panic disorder, depression, and social anxiety [49]. Stanley et al. [102] assessed 254 female firefighters and found anxiety sensitivity to be a significant predictor of suicide risk.

Although anxiety sensitivity has been shown to predict symptoms of mental health in firefighters, the relationship is reciprocal. Specifically, PTSD symptom severity in female firefighters significantly predicted the individual difference factor of anxiety sensitivity [102]. This has potentially important implications for firefighters as both a screening tool and a specific target for interventions. Given that firefighters with elevated anxiety sensitivity are at an increased risk of experiencing PTSD, depression, panic, and social anxiety, it follows that interventions to decrease anxiety sensitivity would decrease these risk factors. Alternatively, interventions that decrease specific risk factors of anxiety sensitivity (e.g., PTSD symptoms) could have large implications on the overall mental health of firefighters.

Insomnia and anxiety sensitivity have been strongly linked in multiple studies [103–105]. Kim et al. [106] assessed 95 mentally healthy adults in the general population of Korea to determine the relationship between insomnia severity and anxiety sensitivity as well as other mental health conditions. They found that insomnia severity was significantly correlated with anxiety sensitivity, as well as depression, and anxiety. In a randomized clinical trial, the efficacy of treating anxiety sensitivity on reducing insomnia symptoms was investigated in 151 patients. The findings demonstrated that computerized treatment for anxiety sensitivity resulted in significant reductions in insomnia symptoms at three- and six-month follow-up periods, even when controlling for reductions in depression and anxiety [107].

4.2. Emotional Regulation and Emotional Intelligence

Emotional regulation and intelligence have also been examined as potential mediating factors explaining the relationship between mental health and insomnia. Emotional regulation is an individual difference trait that explains, to some degree, the level of control an individual has over their emotions. Specifically, in a given situation, emotional regulation can affect the intensity, duration, and type of emotion exhibited [108]. Individuals living with significant mental health symptoms associated with depression, anxiety, and/or PTSD (to name a few) may experience an impairment in emotion regulation. Thus, individuals are at an increased risk of encountering negative emotional states and are less equipped to effectively cope with them, leading to decreased sleep quality and insomnia [30]. On the other hand, individuals with higher emotional intelligence display an increase in psychological well-being [109]. Emotional intelligence highlights an individual's ability to recognize their emotions and the emotions of those around them, label these emotions effectively, and use this information to make rational decisions [110,111]. As established above, firefighters are exposed to significantly greater levels of occupational stress. Emotional intelligence has been shown to indirectly influence perceived stress [112], thus individuals with higher emotional intelligence may experience a blunted stress response or decreased distress during traumatic events.

Daily emotional distress is regulated during REM sleep as limbic activation during REM sleep reactivates emotionally distressing events, associates them with previous occurrences, and then processes them [113]. Restless or fragmented REM sleep interferes with the process of distress resolution thereby contributing to a state of chronic hyperarousal, which is a primary symptom of insomnia [114,115]. Interestingly, Wassing et al. [27] demonstrated that maladaptive sleep periods associated with insomnia may worsen the traumatic exposures compared to those without insomnia; thus, instead of sleep resolving emotional distress, the maladaptive sleep periods increased the distress. Emotional regulation has been associated with numerous mental health disorders and has often been used to explain how specific conditions are related. In trauma-exposed firefighters, emotional regulation has shown a significant relationship with PTSD and depression [49]. As mentioned above, there is evidence linking PTSD symptom severity and the use of alcohol as a coping mechanism specifically in firefighters. Recent evidence suggests emotional regulation may explain the association between PTSD symptom severity and alcohol use as a coping mechanism in firefighters [116].

4.3. Distress Tolerance

Another factor that has shown promise with regards to the amelioration of mental health symptoms is distress tolerance. Distress tolerance is an individual difference trait that provides a self-report measure for an individual's perceived capability to manage negative emotional states [117]. Lower distress tolerance scores have been associated with significant mental health concerns.

While previous research highlights the increased risk of suicide among firefighters exposed to greater occupational stress, the recent literature has found firefighters with higher distress tolerance attenuated this increased risk [55]. Further, due to increased occupational stress, firefighters are at a significantly greater risk to seek negative external coping mechanisms. Substance abuse has been reported by over half of professional firefighters [7]. However, it appears as though higher distress tolerance may reduce the risk of alcohol abuse among firefighters. In a sample of 652 trauma-exposed firefighters, distress tolerance was significantly related to alcohol abuse and other coping motives [118]. It follows logically that individuals with greater depressive symptomology experience negative emotional states more frequently. However, Yoon et al. [119] conducted a meta-analysis on distress tolerance and depression. Their results indicate a systematic relationship between lower distress tolerance and depression. That is, individuals with greater distress tolerance were less likely to display symptoms of depression. Distress tolerance has been negatively associated with numerous other mental health concerns, including PTSD [120] and anxiety [121].

Like emotional regulation, distress tolerance is associated with sleep quality. In a sample of military veterans, perceived sleep quality was positively associated with a self-reported distress tolerance with a poorer sleep relating to reduced distress tolerance as well as increased frustration in a distressing task [122]. Smith et al. [123] examined the association of sleep disturbance and distress tolerance in 652 firefighters and found that 48.6% had disturbed sleep and lower distress tolerance was significantly associated with greater sleep disturbance. To determine the best forms of treatment, the mechanisms linking distress tolerance, emotional regulation, and anxiety sensitivity to sleep quality warrant further investigation.

5. Sleep and Mental Health Interventions in Firefighters

5.1. Current Interventions

There is a need for interventions in full-time firefighters to determine applicable and successful strategies to improve their sleep quality and/or aspects of mental health. Table 1 summarizes the outcomes of various mental health and sleep interventions in full-time firefighters. Other intervention-based studies do exist; however, they are not specific to full-time firefighters but rather recruit firefighters (individuals employed by fire departments prior to becoming a full-time firefighter) or first responders (police, firefighters, EMS) [124–126]. It is important to specifically assess intervention outcomes for full-time firefighters as their schedule, trauma exposure, and occupational requirements are different than other first responders and recruit firefighters.

Table 1. Mental health and sleep interventions in full-time firefighters.

Study	Participants and Intervention	Outcome Measure(s)	Summary of Findings
Jang et al. (2020) [127], Korea	Participants: 39 firefighters Intervention: Single-group pre–post study design; utilized the Firefighter's Therapy for Insomnia and Nightmares (FIT-IN) program which included two 90 min face-to-face group sessions and one 20 min individual phone session with a therapist for brief behavioral therapy for insomnia combined with imagery rehearsal.	•Insomnia severity index (ISI) •Disturbing dream and nightmare severity index (DDNSI) •Epworth Sleepiness Scale (ESS) •Depressive symptom inventory-suicidality subscale (DSI) •Patient Health Questionnaire-9 (PHQ-9) •Two-week sleep diary	The FIT-IN program resulted in a significant increase in sleep efficiency and decrease in sleep onset latency, the number of awakenings, and time in bed as well as insomnia and nightmare severity. Additionally, there were significant improvements in PTSD symptoms, depression, and daytime sleepiness.
Barger et al. (2016) [128], United States	Participants: 6101 firefighters Intervention: Firefighters were placed into a sleep health program (SHP) that provided a sleep health education training session with one of three delivery approaches: expert-led, train-the-trainer, or online.	•Screening for sleep disorders •Assessment of the sleep health educational material One-year follow-up on sleep	The expert-led delivery method of the SHP had the highest participation rate, highest assessment scores, and showed a greater number of firefighters seeking help for sleep disorders than the train-the-trainer and online delivery SHP approaches.
Mehrdad et al. (2015) [129], Iran	Participants: 27 firefighters with poor sleep quality Intervention: In a double-blind, randomized, placebo-controlled crossover trial, firefighters took 10 mg of zolpidem (sleeping pill) for two weeks and a placebo for two weeks with a two-week washout period between conditions.	•Persian version of the Pittsburgh Sleep Quality Index (PSQI)	There was a significant improvement in PSQI scores after the zolpidem period compared to the control period including improved sleep quality, sleep onset latency, sleep duration, habitual sleep efficiency, sleep disturbances, and daytime dysfunction.
Sullivan et al. (2017) [130], United States	Participants: 1189 firefighters Intervention: Firefighters attended a 30 min sleep health education training; those that attended the training were in the intervention group (n = 560), and those that did not attend the training were considered the control group (n = 629).	•Screening for sleep disorders •Firefighter health (sick time) and safety (motor vehicle crashes and injuries) were assessed from departmental records during the study's two-week period •Baseline and end-of-year surveys on subjective improvements in sleep and general health	Firefighters that attended the sleep health education training were 24% less likely to file an official injury report during the study period than those in the control group. There were no changes in self-reported sleep, departmental injury, or motor vehicle crash rates between the groups during the study period.

5.2. Suggested Intervention: Regular Exercise

Future interventional studies should assess the effects of regular exercise on both sleep quality and mental health in firefighters. A large amount of evidence exists that supports the efficacy of chronic exercise for improving subjective sleep quality in individuals suffering from insomnia symptoms. Multiple meta-analytic reviews have investigated exercise interventions on sleep quality and demonstrated overall significant improvements, especially in subjective sleep complaints [131–135]. In a meta-analysis on exercise as an alternative treatment for chronic insomnia, Passos et al. found that the efficacy of chronic exercise was similar to hypnotic drug use in improving symptoms of insomnia [131]. Multiple types of chronic exercise, from aerobic exercise to Tai Chi, have been shown to improve sleep [132]. Several mechanisms that provide a rationale for the improvement in insomnia symptoms from exercise have been suggested [133,136–139]; these include but are not limited to reducing core body temperature for sleep onset [140–143], increasing melatonin and serotonin secretion [131,144], reducing depression and anxiety, and improving autonomic regulation which may reduce hyperarousal associated with insomnia [143].

Exercise also has a strong history of alleviating symptoms of mental health disorders; it is often used as a stand-alone treatment method as well as in conjunction with traditional treatment methods for specific mental health conditions. A recent meta-analysis and systematic review support the use of aerobic exercise as an effective intervention (i.e., large or moderate-to-large effects) to alleviate the symptoms of depression in clinically depressed individuals [145]. Aylett et al. [146] conducted a systematic review and meta-analysis on exercise and anxiety. Their results indicate exercise to be effective at reducing anxiety in individuals diagnosed with anxiety disorders and individuals who self-report elevated anxiety. Additionally, the evidence suggests high-intensity exercise to be more effective at reducing anxiety, but both high- and low-intensity exercise were significantly more effective relative to no exercise [146]. While the effects of exercise on PTSD are still being explored, numerous studies highlight the positive benefits of exercise on PTSD. A recent review and meta-analysis have highlighted the beneficial effects of exercise on PTSD symptoms and some comorbid symptoms. Specifically, exercise reduced PTSD symptom severity and reduced substance abuse [147]. Vancampfort et al. [148] conducted a systematic review and meta-analysis on physical activity and suicidal ideation. While the results are based on cross-sectional data, there was a significant negative association between physical activity and suicidal ideation. Further, individuals who reported meeting current physical activity guidelines were significantly less likely to report suicidal ideation, while individuals who did not meet current physical activity guidelines were significantly more likely to report suicidal ideation [148].

While this is not a comprehensive list, the effects of exercise on mental health disorders, symptomology, and comorbid conditions have been well established. As mentioned above, anxiety, depression, PTSD, substance abuse, and suicidal ideation are often experienced together but remain independent of one another (i.e., not caused by each other). Implementing a single intervention to treat multiple mental health conditions may be challenging as each condition should be evaluated separately. However, exercise appears to have significant positive effects on all the mental health conditions described in this review.

6. Conclusions

Firefighters are at a greater risk for insomnia and mental health conditions due to their shift-working schedules, continual loud alerting emergency alarms, regular psychological and physical trauma exposure, and extreme occupational demands compared to the general population. In addition, sleep and mental health impairments are cyclical as both have been shown to affect the other. Therefore, it is of the utmost importance to determine the best strategies to improve these impairments in full-time firefighters in hopes of leading to a higher quality of life throughout their career as the community relies on their help. In addition, it is important for clinicians that work with firefighters, or other related occupations, to understand the cyclical relationship between insomnia and mental health conditions to better identify appropriate treatment strategies. Due to the supporting evidence, exercise as a treatment for insomnia and mental health conditions in firefighters should be further explored. Exercise interventions should assess multiple modes and intensities of exercise in addition to adherence rates to best determine the most effective and applicable type of regular exercise program to promote in fire departments.

Author Contributions: Conceptualization, A.M.H.-W. and D.R.G.; writing—original draft preparation, A.M.H.-W., D.R.G. and T.J.O.; writing—review and editing, A.M.H.-W., D.R.G. and T.J.O.; supervision, A.M.H.-W. All authors have read and agreed to the published version of the manuscript.

Funding: This research received no external funding.

Institutional Review Board Statement: Not applicable.

Informed Consent Statement: Not applicable.

Data Availability Statement: No new data were created or analyzed in this study. Data sharing is not applicable to this article.

Conflicts of Interest: The authors declare no conflict of interest.

References

1. Carleton, R.N.; Afifi, T.O.; Taillieu, T.; Turner, S.; Krakauer, R.; Anderson, G.S.; MacPhee, R.S.; Ricciardelli, R.; Cramm, H.A.; Groll, D. Exposures to potentially traumatic events among public safety personnel in Canada. *Can. J. Behav. Sci./Rev. Can. Sci. Comport.* **2019**, *51*, 37. [CrossRef]
2. Fraess-Phillips, A.; Wagner, S.; Harris, R.L. Firefighters and traumatic stress: A review. *Int. J. Emerg. Serv.* **2017**, *6*, 67–80. [CrossRef]
3. Harvey, S.B.; Milligan-Saville, J.S.; Paterson, H.M.; Harkness, E.L.; Marsh, A.M.; Dobson, M.; Kemp, R.; Bryant, R.A. The mental health of fire-fighters: An examination of the impact of repeated trauma exposure. *Aust. N. Z. J. Psychiatry* **2016**, *50*, 649–658. [CrossRef] [PubMed]
4. Jahnke, S.A.; Poston, W.S.C.; Haddock, C.K.; Murphy, B. Firefighting and mental health: Experiences of repeated exposure to trauma. *Work* **2016**, *53*, 737–744. [CrossRef] [PubMed]
5. Marciniak, R.A.; Tesch, C.J.; Ebersole, K.T. Heart rate response to alarm tones in firefighters. *Int. Arch. Occup. Environ. Health* **2021**, *94*, 783–789. [CrossRef]
6. Paterson, J.L.; Aisbett, B.; Ferguson, S.A. Sound the alarm: Health and safety risks associated with alarm response for salaried and retained metropolitan firefighters. *Saf. Sci.* **2016**, *82*, 174–181. [CrossRef]
7. Carey, M.G.; Al-Zaiti, S.S.; Dean, G.E.; Sessanna, L.; Finnell, D.S. Sleep problems, depression, substance use, social bonding, and quality of life in professional firefighters. *J. Occup. Environ. Med.* **2011**, *53*, 928–933. [CrossRef]
8. Jalilian, H.; Ziaei, M.; Weiderpass, E.; Rueegg, C.S.; Khosravi, Y.; Kjaerheim, K. Cancer incidence and mortality among firefighters. *Int. J. Cancer* **2019**, *145*, 2639–2646. [CrossRef]
9. Soteriades, E.S.; Smith, D.L.; Tsismenakis, A.J.; Baur, D.M.; Kales, S.N. Cardiovascular disease in US firefighters: A systematic review. *Cardiol. Rev.* **2011**, *19*, 202–215. [CrossRef]
10. Cramm, H.; Richmond, R.; Jamshidi, L.; Edgelow, M.; Groll, D.; Ricciardelli, R.; MacDermid, J.C.; Keiley, M.; Carleton, R.N. Mental Health of Canadian Firefighters: The Impact of Sleep. *Int. J. Environ. Res. Public Health* **2021**, *18*, 13256. [CrossRef]
11. Billings, J.; Focht, W. Firefighter Shift Schedules Affect Sleep Quality. *J. Occup. Environ. Med.* **2016**, *58*, 294–298. [CrossRef] [PubMed]
12. Choi, B.; Schnall, P.L.; Dobson, M.; Garcia-Rivas, J.; Kim, H.; Zaldivar, F.; Israel, L.; Baker, D. Very Long (>48 hours) Shifts and Cardiovascular Strain in Firefighters: A Theoretical Framework. *Ann. Occup. Environ. Med.* **2014**, *26*, 5. [CrossRef] [PubMed]
13. Blau, G. Exploring the impact of sleep-related impairments on the perceived general health and retention intent of an Emergency Medical Services (EMS) sample. *Career Dev. Int.* **2011**, *16*, 238–253. [CrossRef]
14. Zhu, L.; Zee, P.C. Circadian rhythm sleep disorders. *Neurol. Clin.* **2012**, *30*, 1167–1191. [CrossRef] [PubMed]
15. Klerman, E.B. Clinical aspects of human circadian rhythms. *J. Biol. Rhythm.* **2005**, *20*, 375–386. [CrossRef] [PubMed]
16. Vargas de Barros, V.; Martins, L.F.; Saitz, R.; Bastos, R.R.; Ronzani, T.M. Mental health conditions, individual and job characteristics and sleep disturbances among firefighters. *J. Health Psychol.* **2013**, *18*, 350–358. [CrossRef] [PubMed]
17. Watson, N.F.; Badr, M.S.; Belenky, G.; Bliwise, D.L.; Buxton, O.M.; Buysse, D.; Dinges, D.F.; Gangwisch, J.; Grandner, M.A.; Kushida, C.; et al. Recommended Amount of Sleep for a Healthy Adult: A Joint Consensus Statement of the American Academy of Sleep Medicine and Sleep Research Society. *Sleep* **2015**, *38*, 843–844. [CrossRef]
18. McCarley, R.W. Neurobiology of REM and NREM sleep. *Sleep Med.* **2007**, *8*, 302–330. [CrossRef] [PubMed]
19. Baran, B.; Pace-Schott, E.F.; Ericson, C.; Spencer, R.M. Processing of emotional reactivity and emotional memory over sleep. *J. Neurosci.* **2012**, *32*, 1035–1042. [CrossRef]
20. Van der Helm, E.; Walker, M.P. Sleep and emotional memory processing. *Sleep Med. Clin.* **2011**, *6*, 31–43. [CrossRef]
21. Hutchison, I.C.; Rathore, S. The role of REM sleep theta activity in emotional memory. *Front. Psychol.* **2015**, *6*, 1439. [CrossRef] [PubMed]

22. Vyazovskiy, V.V.; Delogu, A. NREM and REM sleep: Complementary roles in recovery after wakefulness. *Neuroscientist* **2014**, *20*, 203–219. [CrossRef] [PubMed]
23. Klemm, W. Why does REM sleep occur? A wake-up hypothesis. *Front. Syst. Neurosci.* **2011**, *5*, 73. [CrossRef] [PubMed]
24. Roth, T. Characteristics and determinants of normal sleep. *J. Clin. Psychiatry* **2004**, *65* (Suppl. 16), 8–11. [PubMed]
25. Léger, D.; Guilleminault, C.; Bader, G.; Lévy, E.; Paillard, M. Medical and socio-professional impact of insomnia. *Sleep* **2002**, *25*, 621–625. [CrossRef]
26. Morin, C.M.; Drake, C.L.; Harvey, A.G.; Krystal, A.D.; Manber, R.; Riemann, D.; Spiegelhalder, K. Insomnia disorder. *Nat. Rev. Dis. Primers* **2015**, *1*, 15026. [CrossRef] [PubMed]
27. Wassing, R.; Benjamins, J.S.; Talamini, L.M.; Schalkwijk, F.; Van Someren, E.J. Overnight worsening of emotional distress indicates maladaptive sleep in insomnia. *Sleep* **2019**, *42*, zsy268. [CrossRef] [PubMed]
28. Germain, A.; Buysse, D.J.; Nofzinger, E. Sleep-specific mechanisms underlying posttraumatic stress disorder: Integrative review and neurobiological hypotheses. *Sleep Med. Rev.* **2008**, *12*, 185–195. [CrossRef] [PubMed]
29. Corneil, W.; Beaton, R.; Murphy, S.; Johnson, C.; Pike, K. Exposure to traumatic incidents and prevalence of posttraumatic stress symptomatology in urban firefighters in two countries. *J. Occup. Health Psychol.* **1999**, *4*, 131–141. [CrossRef]
30. Hom, M.A.; Stanley, I.H.; Rogers, M.L.; Tzoneva, M.; Bernert, R.A.; Joiner, T.E. The association between sleep disturbances and depression among firefighters: Emotion dysregulation as an explanatory factor. *J. Clin. Sleep Med.* **2016**, *12*, 235–245. [CrossRef]
31. Wolffe, T.A.M.; Robinson, A.; Clinton, A.; Turrell, L.; Stec, A.A. Mental health of UK firefighters. *Sci. Rep.* **2023**, *13*, 62. [CrossRef] [PubMed]
32. Roth, T. Insomnia: Definition, prevalence, etiology, and consequences. *J. Clin. Sleep Med.* **2007**, *3* (Suppl. 5), S7–S10. [CrossRef] [PubMed]
33. Vargas, I.; Nguyen, A.M.; Muench, A.; Bastien, C.H.; Ellis, J.G.; Perlis, M.L. Acute and chronic insomnia: What has time and/or hyperarousal got to do with it? *Brain Sci.* **2020**, *10*, 71. [CrossRef]
34. Harvey, A.G. Insomnia: Symptom or diagnosis? *Clin. Psychol. Rev.* **2001**, *21*, 1037–1059. [CrossRef]
35. Sateia, M.J. International classification of sleep disorders. *Chest* **2014**, *146*, 1387–1394. [CrossRef]
36. Schutte-Rodin, S.; Broch, L.; Buysse, D.; Dorsey, C.; Sateia, M. Clinical guideline for the evaluation and management of chronic insomnia in adults. *J. Clin. Sleep Med.* **2008**, *4*, 487–504. [CrossRef]
37. Ohayon, M.M. Epidemiology of insomnia: What we know and what we still need to learn. *Sleep Med. Rev.* **2002**, *6*, 97–111. [CrossRef]
38. Ohayon, M.M.; Reynolds, C.F. III. Epidemiological and clinical relevance of insomnia diagnosis algorithms according to the DSM-IV and the International Classification of Sleep Disorders (ICSD). *Sleep Med.* **2009**, *10*, 952–960. [CrossRef] [PubMed]
39. Roth, T.; Jaeger, S.; Jin, R.; Kalsekar, A.; Stang, P.E.; Kessler, R.C. Sleep problems, comorbid mental disorders, and role functioning in the national comorbidity survey replication. *Biol. Psychiatry* **2006**, *60*, 1364–1371. [CrossRef]
40. Buysse, D.J.; Reynolds, C.F., 3rd; Monk, T.H.; Berman, S.R.; Kupfer, D.J. The Pittsburgh Sleep Quality Index: A new instrument for psychiatric practice and research. *Psychiatry Res.* **1989**, *28*, 193–213. [CrossRef]
41. Walker, N.A.; Sunderram, J.; Zhang, P.; Lu S-e Scharf, M.T. Clinical utility of the Epworth sleepiness scale. *Sleep Breath.* **2020**, *24*, 1759–1765. [CrossRef] [PubMed]
42. Bastien, C.H.; Vallières, A.; Morin, C.M. Validation of the Insomnia Severity Index as an outcome measure for insomnia research. *Sleep Med.* **2001**, *2*, 297–307. [CrossRef] [PubMed]
43. Mehrdad, R.; Haghighi, K.S.; Esfahani, A.H. Sleep quality of professional firefighters. *Int. J. Prev. Med.* **2013**, *4*, 1095–1100.
44. Lim, D.-K.; Baek, K.-O.; Chung, I.-S.; Lee, M.-Y. Factors related to sleep disorders among male firefighters. *Ann. Occup. Environ. Med.* **2014**, *26*, 1–8. [CrossRef]
45. Asghari, A.; Farhadi, M.; Kamrava, S.K.; Ghalehbaghi, B.; Nojomi, M. Subjective sleep quality in urban population. *Arch. Iran. Med.* **2012**, *15*, 95–98. [PubMed]
46. Wagner, S.L.; White, N.; Buys, N.; Carey, M.G.; Corneil, W.; Fyfe, T.; Matthews, L.R.; Randall, C.; Regehr, C.; White, M.; et al. Systematic review of mental health symptoms in firefighters exposed to routine duty-related critical incidents. *Traumatology* **2021**, *27*, 285–302. [CrossRef]
47. American Psychiatric Association of Mental Disorders. *Diagnostic and Statistical Manual of Mental Disorders: DSM-5™*, 5th ed.; American Psychiatric Publishing, Inc.: Washington, DC, USA, 2013. [CrossRef]
48. Selye, H. *Stress in Health and Disease*; Butterworth-Heinemann: Oxford, UK, 2013.
49. Paulus, D.J.; Gallagher, M.W.; Bartlett, B.A.; Tran, J.; Vujanovic, A.A. The unique and interactive effects of anxiety sensitivity and emotion dysregulation in relation to posttraumatic stress, depressive, and anxiety symptoms among trauma-exposed firefighters. *Compr. Psychiatry* **2018**, *84*, 54–61. [CrossRef]
50. CareerCast. Most Stressful Jobs of 2017. 2017. Available online: http://www.careercast.com/jobs-rated/most-stressful-jobs-2017 (accessed on 10 February 2024).
51. Wiegand, D.M.; Chiu, S. *Evaluation of Fire Fighters' Mental Health Symptoms and Exposure to Traumatic Events, Job Stress, and Bloodborne Pathogens*; Centers for Disease Control and Prevention: Cincinnati, OH, USA, 2017. Available online: https://www.cdc.gov/niosh/hhe/reports/pdfs/2017-0021-3293.pdf (accessed on 10 February 2024).

52. Huang, G.; Chu, H.; Chen, R.; Liu, D.; Banda, K.J.; O'Brien, A.P.; Jen, H.J.; Chiang, K.J.; Chiou, J.F.; Chou, K.R. Prevalence of depression, anxiety, and stress among first responders for medical emergencies during COVID-19 pandemic: A meta-analysis. *J. Glob. Health* **2022**, *12*, 05028. [CrossRef]
53. Meyer, E.C.; Zimering, R.; Daly, E.; Knight, J.; Kamholz, B.W.; Gulliver, S.B. Predictors of posttraumatic stress disorder and other psychological symptoms in trauma-exposed firefighters. *Psychol. Serv.* **2012**, *9*, 1–15. [CrossRef]
54. Sawhney, G.; Jennings, K.S.; Britt, T.W.; Sliter, M.T. Occupational stress and mental health symptoms: Examining the moderating effect of work recovery strategies in firefighters. *J. Occup. Health Psychol.* **2018**, *23*, 443. [CrossRef]
55. Stanley, I.H.; Boffa, J.W.; Smith, L.J.; Tran, J.K.; Schmidt, N.B.; Joiner, T.E.; Vujanovic, A.A. Occupational stress and suicidality among firefighters: Examining the buffering role of distress tolerance. *Psychiatry Res.* **2018**, *266*, 90–96. [CrossRef] [PubMed]
56. Yook, Y.S. Firefighters' occupational stress and its correlations with cardiorespiratory fitness, arterial stiffness, heart rate variability and sleep quality. *PLoS ONE* **2019**, *14*, e0226739. [CrossRef] [PubMed]
57. Bromet, E.; Andrade, L.H.; Hwang, I.; Sampson, N.A.; Alonso, J.; de Girolamo, G.; de Graaf, R.; Demyttenaere, K.; Hu, C.; Iwata N.; et al. Cross-national epidemiology of DSM-IV major depressive episode. *BMC Med.* **2011**, *9*, 90. [CrossRef] [PubMed]
58. Fullerton, C.S.; Ursano, R.J.; Wang, L. Acute stress disorder, posttraumatic stress disorder, and depression in disaster or rescue workers. *Am. J. Psychiatry* **2004**, *161*, 1370–1376. [CrossRef]
59. Kessler, R.C.; Merikangas, K.R.; Wang, P.S. Prevalence, comorbidity, and service utilization for mood disorders in the United States at the beginning of the twenty-first century. *Annu. Rev. Clin. Psychol.* **2007**, *3*, 137–158. [CrossRef]
60. Hasin, D.S.; Goodwin, R.D.; Stinson, F.S.; Grant, B.F. Epidemiology of major depressive disorder: Results from the National Epidemiologic Survey on Alcoholism and Related Conditions. *Arch. Gen. Psychiatry* **2005**, *62*, 1097–1106. [CrossRef] [PubMed]
61. Nock, M.K.; Hwang, I.; Sampson, N.A.; Kessler, R.C. Mental disorders, comorbidity and suicidal behavior: Results from the National Comorbidity Survey Replication. *Mol. Psychiatry* **2010**, *15*, 868–876. [CrossRef]
62. Alghamdi, M.; Hunt, N.; Thomas, S. Prevalence rate of PTSD, depression and anxiety symptoms among Saudi firefighters. *J. Trauma. Stress Disord. Treat.* **2016**, *6*, 2. [CrossRef]
63. Baglioni, C.; Battagliese, G.; Feige, B.; Spiegelhalder, K.; Nissen, C.; Voderholzer, U.; Lombardo, C.; Riemann, D. Insomnia as a predictor of depression: A meta-analytic evaluation of longitudinal epidemiological studies. *J. Affect. Disord.* **2011**, *135*, 10–19. [CrossRef]
64. Heinrichs, M.; Wagner, D.; Schoch, W.; Soravia, L.M.; Hellhammer, D.H.; Ehlert, U. Predicting posttraumatic stress symptoms from pretraumatic risk factors: A 2-year prospective follow-up study in firefighters. *Am. J. Psychiatry* **2005**, *162*, 2276–2286. [CrossRef]
65. Katsavouni, F.; Bebetsos, E.; Malliou, P.; Beneka, A. The relationship between burnout, PTSD symptoms and injuries in firefighters. *Occup. Med.* **2016**, *66*, 32–37. [CrossRef] [PubMed]
66. Obuobi-Donkor, G.; Oluwasina, F.; Nkire, N.; Agyapong, V.I.O. A Scoping Review on the Prevalence and Determinants of Post-Traumatic Stress Disorder among Military Personnel and Firefighters: Implications for Public Policy and Practice. *Int. J. Environ. Res. Public Health* **2022**, *19*, 1565. [CrossRef] [PubMed]
67. Rosellini, A.J.; Heeringa, S.G.; Stein, M.B.; Ursano, R.J.; Chiu, W.T.; Colpe, L.J.; Fullerton, C.S.; Gilman, S.E.; Hwang, I.; Naifeh J.A.; et al. Lifetime prevalence of DSM-IV mental disorders among new soldiers in the U.S. Army: Results from the Army Study to Assess Risk and Resilience in Servicemembers (Army STARRS). *Depress. Anxiety* **2015**, *32*, 13–24. [CrossRef] [PubMed]
68. Elhai, J.D.; Grubaugh, A.L.; Kashdan, T.B.; Frueh, B.C. Empirical examination of a proposed refinement to DSM-IV posttraumatic stress disorder symptom criteria using the National Comorbidity Survey Replication data. *J. Clin. Psychiatry* **2008**, *69*, 597. [CrossRef]
69. Bing-Canar, H.; Ranney, R.M.; McNett, S.; Tran, J.K.; Berenz, E.C.; Vujanovic, A.A. Alcohol Use Problems, Posttraumatic Stress Disorder, and Suicide Risk among Trauma-Exposed Firefighters. *J. Nerv. Ment. Dis.* **2019**, *207*, 192–198. [CrossRef] [PubMed]
70. Salleh, M.N.B.M.; Ismail, H.B.; Yusoff, H.B.M. Prevalence and predictors for PTSD among firefighters. A systematic review. *Int. J. Public Health Res.* **2020**, *10*.
71. Davidson, J.R.; Rothbaum, B.O.; van der Kolk, B.A.; Sikes, C.R.; Farfel, G.M. Multicenter, double-blind comparison of sertraline and placebo in the treatment of posttraumatic stress disorder. *Arch. Gen. Psychiatry* **2001**, *58*, 485–492. [CrossRef]
72. Zayfert, C.; DeViva, J.C. Residual insomnia following cognitive behavioral therapy for PTSD. *J. Trauma. Stress Off. Publ. Int. Soc Trauma. Stress Stud.* **2004**, *17*, 69–73. [CrossRef] [PubMed]
73. Mohammadi, M.R.; Ghanizadeh, A.; Rahgozar, M.; Noorbala, A.A.; Davidian, H.; Afzali, H.M.; Naghavi, H.R.; Yazdi, S.A.B. Saberi, S.M.; Mesgarpour, B. Prevalence of obsessive-compulsive disorder in Iran. *BMC Psychiatry* **2004**, *4*, 2. [CrossRef]
74. Fawcett, E.J.; Power, H.; Fawcett, J.M. Women are at greater risk of OCD than men: A meta-analytic review of OCD prevalence worldwide. *J. Clin. Psychiatry* **2020**, *81*, 13075. [CrossRef]
75. Haynes, H.J.; Stein, G.P. *US Fire Department Profile 2015*; National Fire Protection Association: Quincy, MA, USA, 2017.
76. Hofer, P.D.; Wahl, K.; Meyer, A.H.; Miché, M.; Beesdo-Baum, K.; Wong, S.F.; Grisham, J.R.; Wittchen, H.U.; Lieb, R. Obsessive-compulsive disorder and the risk of subsequent mental disorders: A community study of adolescents and young adults. *Depress. Anxiety* **2018**, *35*, 339–345. [CrossRef] [PubMed]
77. Angelakis, I.; Gooding, P.; Tarrier, N.; Panagioti, M. Suicidality in obsessive compulsive disorder (OCD): A systematic review and meta-analysis. *Clin. Psychol. Rev.* **2015**, *39*, 1–15. [CrossRef] [PubMed]

78. Bradley, D.J. The Physiological Effects of Firefighters in Response to the Duality of Heat and Emergency Crises. *Int. J. Public Priv. Perspect. Healthc. Cult. Environ. (IJPPPHCE)* **2022**, *6*, 1–15. [CrossRef]
79. Stanley, I.H.; Hom, M.A.; Joiner, T.E. A systematic review of suicidal thoughts and behaviors among police officers, firefighters, EMTs, and paramedics. *Clin. Psychol. Rev.* **2016**, *44*, 25–44. [CrossRef] [PubMed]
80. Kessler, R.C.; Borges, G.; Walters, E.E. Prevalence of and risk factors for lifetime suicide attempts in the National Comorbidity Survey. *Arch. Gen. Psychiatry* **1999**, *56*, 617–626. [CrossRef] [PubMed]
81. Stanley, I.H.; Hom, M.A.; Hagan, C.R.; Joiner, T.E. Career prevalence and correlates of suicidal thoughts and behaviors among firefighters. *J. Affect. Disord.* **2015**, *187*, 163–171. [CrossRef] [PubMed]
82. World Health Organization. *Preventing Suicide: A Global Imperative*; World Health Organization: Geneva, Switzerland, 2014.
83. Cougle, J.R.; Keough, M.E.; Riccardi, C.J.; Sachs-Ericsson, N. Anxiety disorders and suicidality in the National Comorbidity Survey-Replication. *J. Psychiatr. Res.* **2009**, *43*, 825–829. [CrossRef] [PubMed]
84. Boffa, J.W.; Stanley, I.H.; Hom, M.A.; Norr, A.M.; Joiner, T.E.; Schmidt, N.B. PTSD symptoms and suicidal thoughts and behaviors among firefighters. *J. Psychiatr. Res.* **2017**, *84*, 277–283. [CrossRef] [PubMed]
85. Martin, C.E.; Tran, J.K.; Buser, S.J. Correlates of suicidality in firefighter/EMS personnel. *J. Affect. Disord.* **2017**, *208*, 177–183. [CrossRef]
86. Goodwin, R.D.; Marusic, A. Association between short sleep and suicidal ideation and suicide attempt among adults in the general population. *Sleep* **2008**, *31*, 1097–1101.
87. Krahn, L.E.; Miller, B.W.; Bergstrom, L.R. Rapid resolution of intense suicidal ideation after treatment of severe obstructive sleep apnea. *J. Clin. Sleep Med.* **2008**, *4*, 64–65. [CrossRef] [PubMed]
88. Haddock, C.K.; Jitnarin, N.; Caetano, R.; Jahnke, S.A.; Hollerbach, B.S.; Kaipust, C.M.; Poston, W.S. Norms about alcohol use among US firefighters. *Saf. Health Work* **2022**, *13*, 387–393. [CrossRef] [PubMed]
89. Grucza, R.A.; Sher, K.J.; Kerr, W.C.; Krauss, M.J.; Lui, C.K.; McDowell, Y.E.; Hartz, S.; Virdi, G.; Bierut, L.J. Trends in adult alcohol use and binge drinking in the early 21st-century United States: A meta-analysis of 6 National Survey Series. *Alcohol Clin. Exp. Res.* **2018**, *42*, 1939–1950. [CrossRef] [PubMed]
90. Haddock, C.K.; Poston, W.S.C.; Jahnke, S.A.; Jitnarin, N. Alcohol Use and Problem Drinking among Women Firefighters. *Womens Health Issues* **2017**, *27*, 632–638. [CrossRef] [PubMed]
91. Jahnke, S.A.; Poston, W.S.; Haddock, C.K.; Jitnarin, N.; Hyder, M.L.; Horvath, C. The health of women in the US fire service. *BMC Womens Health* **2012**, *12*, 39. [CrossRef] [PubMed]
92. Azevedo, D.S.d.S.d.; Lima, E.D.P.; Assunção, A.Á. Factors associated with the use of anxiolytic drugs among military firefighters. *Rev. Bras. Epidemiol.* **2019**, *22*, e190021. [CrossRef] [PubMed]
93. Rasmus, P.; Kocur, J.; Flirski, M.; Sobów, T. Biopsychosocial correlates of psychoactive substance use in professional firefighters. *J. Med. Sci. Technol.* **2013**, *54*, 70–75.
94. Bartlett, B.A.; Smith, L.J.; Lebeaut, A.; Tran, J.K.; Vujanovic, A.A. PTSD symptom severity and impulsivity among firefighters: Associations with alcohol use. *Psychiatry Res.* **2019**, *278*, 315–323. [CrossRef] [PubMed]
95. Pfefferbaum, B.; North, C.S.; Bunch, K.; Wilson, T.G.; Tucker, P.; Schorr, J.K. The impact of the 1995 Oklahoma City bombing on the partners of firefighters. *J. Urban Health* **2002**, *79*, 364–372. [CrossRef]
96. Bacharach, S.B.; Bamberger, P.A.; Doveh, E. Firefighters, critical incidents, and drinking to cope: The adequacy of unit-level performance resources as a source of vulnerability and protection. *J. Appl. Psychol.* **2008**, *93*, 155. [CrossRef]
97. Martin, C.E.; Vujanovic, A.A.; Paulus, D.J.; Bartlett, B.; Gallagher, M.W.; Tran, J.K. Alcohol use and suicidality in firefighters: Associations with depressive symptoms and posttraumatic stress. *Compr. Psychiatry* **2017**, *74*, 44–52. [CrossRef] [PubMed]
98. Thakkar, M.M.; Sharma, R.; Sahota, P. Alcohol disrupts sleep homeostasis. *Alcohol* **2015**, *49*, 299–310. [CrossRef] [PubMed]
99. Smith, L.J.; Gallagher, M.W.; Tran, J.K.; Vujanovic, A.A. Posttraumatic stress, alcohol use, and alcohol use reasons in firefighters: The role of sleep disturbance. *Compr. Psychiatry* **2018**, *87*, 64–71. [CrossRef] [PubMed]
100. Hunt, C.; Slade, T.; Andrews, G. Generalized anxiety disorder and major depressive disorder comorbidity in the National Survey of Mental Health and Well-Being. *Depress. Anxiety* **2004**, *20*, 23–31. [CrossRef] [PubMed]
101. Taylor, S.; Zvolensky, M.J.; Cox, B.J.; Deacon, B.; Heimberg, R.G.; Ledley, D.R.; Abramowitz, J.S.; Holaway, R.M.; Sandin, B.; Stewart, S.H. Robust dimensions of anxiety sensitivity: Development and initial validation of the Anxiety Sensitivity Index-3. *Psychol. Assess.* **2007**, *19*, 176. [CrossRef] [PubMed]
102. Stanley, I.H.; Hom, M.A.; Spencer-Thomas, S.; Joiner, T.E. Examining anxiety sensitivity as a mediator of the association between PTSD symptoms and suicide risk among women firefighters. *J. Anxiety Disord.* **2017**, *50*, 94–102. [CrossRef] [PubMed]
103. Lauriola, M.; Carleton, R.N.; Tempesta, D.; Calanna, P.; Socci, V.; Mosca, O.; Salfi, F.; De Gennaro, L.; Ferrara, M. A correlational analysis of the relationships among intolerance of uncertainty, anxiety sensitivity, subjective sleep quality, and insomnia symptoms. *Int. J. Environ. Res. Public Health* **2019**, *16*, 3253. [CrossRef] [PubMed]
104. Raines, A.M.; Short, N.A.; Sutton, C.A.; Oglesby, M.E.; Allan, N.P.; Schmidt, N.B. Obsessive-compulsive symptom dimensions and insomnia: The mediating role of anxiety sensitivity cognitive concerns. *Psychiatry Res.* **2015**, *228*, 368–372. [CrossRef]
105. Dixon, L.J.; Lee, A.A.; Gratz, K.L.; Tull, M.T. Anxiety sensitivity and sleep disturbance: Investigating associations among patients with co-occurring anxiety and substance use disorders. *J. Anxiety Disord.* **2018**, *53*, 9–15. [CrossRef]
106. Kim, N.-H.; Choi, H.-M.; Lim, S.-W.; Oh, K.-S. The relationship between insomnia severity and depression, anxiety and anxiety sensitivity in general population. *Sleep Med. Psychophysiol.* **2006**, *13*, 59–66.

107. Short, N.A.; Boffa, J.W.; King, S.; Albanese, B.J.; Allan, N.P.; Schmidt, N.B. A randomized clinical trial examining the effects of an anxiety sensitivity intervention on insomnia symptoms: Replication and extension. *Behav. Res. Ther.* **2017**, *99*, 108–116. [CrossRef] [PubMed]
108. Peña-Sarrionandia, A.; Mikolajczak, M.; Gross, J.J. Integrating emotion regulation and emotional intelligence traditions: A meta-analysis. *Front. Psychol.* **2015**, *6*, 130633. [CrossRef] [PubMed]
109. Salami, S.O. Personality and Psychological Well-Being of Adolescents: The Moderating Role of Emotional Intelligence. *Soc. Behav. Personal. Int. J.* **2011**, *39*, 785–794. [CrossRef]
110. Bușu, A.-F. Emotional intelligence as a type of cognitive ability. *Rev. Științe Politice/Rev. Sci. Polit.* **2020**, *66*, 204–215.
111. Salovey, P.; Mayer, J.D. Emotional intelligence. *Imagin. Cogn. Personal.* **1990**, *9*, 185–211. [CrossRef]
112. Thomas, C.; Zolkoski, S. Preventing stress among undergraduate learners: The importance of emotional intelligence, resilience, and emotion regulation. In *Frontiers in Education*; Frontiers Media SA: Lausanne, Switzerland, 2020.
113. Walker, M.P.; van Der Helm, E. Overnight therapy? The role of sleep in emotional brain processing. *Psychol. Bull.* **2009**, *135*, 731. [CrossRef] [PubMed]
114. Baglioni, C.; Spiegelhalder, K.; Lombardo, C.; Riemann, D. Sleep and emotions: A focus on insomnia. *Sleep Med. Rev.* **2010**, *14*, 227–238. [CrossRef] [PubMed]
115. Wassing, R.; Benjamins, J.S.; Dekker, K.; Moens, S.; Spiegelhalder, K.; Feige, B.; Riemann, D.; van der Sluis, S.; Van Der Werf, Y.D.; Talamini, L.M. Slow dissolving of emotional distress contributes to hyperarousal. *Proc. Natl. Acad. Sci. USA* **2016**, *113*, 2538–2543. [CrossRef]
116. Leonard, S.J.; McGrew, S.J.; Lebeaut, A.; Vujanovic, A.A. PTSD symptom severity and alcohol use among firefighters: The role of emotion regulation difficulties. *J. Dual Diagn.* **2023**, *19*, 209–220. [CrossRef] [PubMed]
117. Simons, J.S.; Gaher, R.M. The Distress Tolerance Scale: Development and validation of a self-report measure. *Motiv. Emot.* **2005**, *29*, 83–102. [CrossRef]
118. Zegel, M.; Tran, J.K.; Vujanovic, A.A. Posttraumatic stress, alcohol use, and alcohol use motives among firefighters: The role of distress tolerance. *Psychiatry Res.* **2019**, *282*, 112633. [CrossRef] [PubMed]
119. Yoon, S.; Dang, V.; Mertz, J.; Rottenberg, J. Are attitudes towards emotions associated with depression? A conceptual and meta-analytic review. *J. Affect. Disord.* **2018**, *232*, 329–340. [CrossRef] [PubMed]
120. Tull, M.; Kimbrel, N. *Emotion in Posttraumatic Stress Disorder: Etiology, Assessment, Neurobiology, and Treatment*; Academic Press: Cambridge, MA, USA, 2020.
121. McHugh, R.K.; Otto, M.W. Refining the measurement of distress intolerance. *Behav. Ther.* **2012**, *43*, 641–651. [CrossRef]
122. Short, N.A.; Babson, K.A.; Schmidt, N.B.; Knight, C.B.; Johnson, J.; Bonn-Miller, M.O. Sleep and affective functioning: Examining the association between sleep quality and distress tolerance among veterans. *Personal. Individ. Differ.* **2016**, *90*, 247–253. [CrossRef]
123. Smith, L.J.; Bartlett, B.A.; Tran, J.K.; Gallagher, M.W.; Alfano, C.; Vujanovic, A.A. Sleep disturbance among firefighters: Understanding associations with alcohol use and distress tolerance. *Cogn. Ther. Res.* **2019**, *43*, 66–77. [CrossRef]
124. Skeffington, P.M.; Rees, C.S.; Mazzucchelli, T.G.; Kane, R.T. The primary prevention of PTSD in firefighters: Preliminary results of an RCT with 12-month follow-up. *PLoS ONE* **2016**, *11*, e0155873. [CrossRef] [PubMed]
125. McKeon, G.; Steel, Z.; Wells, R.; Newby, J.; Hadzi-Pavlovic, D.; Vancampfort, D.; Rosenbaum, S. A mental health–informed physical activity intervention for first responders and their partners delivered using Facebook: Mixed methods pilot study. *JMIR Form. Res.* **2021**, *5*, e23432. [CrossRef]
126. Lan, F.-Y.; Scheibler, C.; Hershey, M.S.; Romero-Cabrera, J.L.; Gaviola, G.C.; Yiannakou, I.; Fernandez-Montero, A.; Christophi, C.A.; Christiani, D.C.; Sotos-Prieto, M. Effects of a healthy lifestyle intervention and COVID-19-adjusted training curriculum on firefighter recruits. *Sci. Rep.* **2022**, *12*, 10607. [CrossRef] [PubMed]
127. Jang, E.H.; Hong, Y.; Kim, Y.; Lee, S.; Ahn, Y.; Jeong, K.S.; Jang, T.-W.; Lim, H.; Jung, E.; Group, S.W.D.S. The development of a sleep intervention for firefighters: The FIT-IN (Firefighter's therapy for insomnia and nightmares) Study. *Int. J. Environ. Res. Public Health* **2020**, *17*, 8738. [CrossRef]
128. Barger, L.K.; O'Brien, C.S.; Rajaratnam, S.M.; Qadri, S.; Sullivan, J.P.; Wang, W.; Czeisler, C.A.; Lockley, S.W. Implementing a sleep health education and sleep disorders screening program in fire departments: A comparison of methodology. *J. Occup. Environ. Med.* **2016**, *58*, 601. [CrossRef]
129. Mehrdad, R.; Haghighi, K.S.; Esfahani, A.H.N. Effect of zolpidem on sleep quality of professional firefighters; a double blind, randomized, placebo-controlled crossover clinical trial. *Acta Medica Iran.* **2015**, *53*, 573–578.
130. Sullivan, J.P.; O'Brien, C.S.; Barger, L.K.; Rajaratnam, S.M.; Czeisler, C.A.; Lockley, S.W.; Harvard Work Hours, H.; Group, S. Randomized, prospective study of the impact of a sleep health program on firefighter injury and disability. *Sleep* **2017**, *40*, zsw001. [CrossRef] [PubMed]
131. Passos, G.S.; Poyares, D.L.R.; Santana, M.G.; Tufik, S.; Mello, M.T.d. Is exercise an alternative treatment for chronic insomnia? *Clinics* **2012**, *67*, 653–660. [CrossRef] [PubMed]
132. D'Aurea, C.V.R.; Frange, C.; Poyares, D.; Souza AAL d Lenza, M. Physical exercise as a therapeutic approach for adults with insomnia: Systematic review and meta-analysis. *Einstein* **2022**, *20*, eAO8058. [CrossRef] [PubMed]
133. Youngstedt, S.D. Effects of exercise on sleep. *Clin. Sports Med.* **2005**, *24*, 355–365. [CrossRef] [PubMed]
134. Kredlow, M.A.; Capozzoli, M.C.; Hearon, B.A.; Calkins, A.W.; Otto, M.W. The effects of physical activity on sleep: A meta-analytic review. *J. Behav. Med.* **2015**, *38*, 427–449. [CrossRef]

35. Banno, M.; Harada, Y.; Taniguchi, M.; Tobita, R.; Tsujimoto, H.; Tsujimoto, Y.; Kataoka, Y.; Noda, A. Exercise can improve sleep quality: A systematic review and meta-analysis. *PeerJ* **2018**, *6*, e5172. [CrossRef]
36. Wang, W.; Sawada, M.; Noriyama, Y.; Arita, K.; Ota, T.; Sadamatsu, M.; Kiyotou, R.; Hirai, M.; Kishimoto, T. Tai Chi exercise versus rehabilitation for the elderly with cerebral vascular disorder: A single-blinded randomized controlled trial. *Psychogeriatrics* **2010**, *10*, 160–166. [CrossRef]
37. Reid, K.J.; Baron, K.G.; Lu, B.; Naylor, E.; Wolfe, L.; Zee, P.C. Aerobic exercise improves self-reported sleep and quality of life in older adults with insomnia. *Sleep Med.* **2010**, *11*, 934–940. [CrossRef]
38. Singh, N.A.; Clements, K.M.; Fiatarone, M.A. A randomized controlled trial of the effect of exercise on sleep. *Sleep* **1997**, *20*, 95–101. [CrossRef]
39. Paluska, S.A.; Schwenk, T.L. Physical activity and mental health: Current concepts. *Sports Med.* **2000**, *29*, 167–180. [CrossRef] [PubMed]
40. Horne, J.; Moore, V. Sleep EEG effects of exercise with and without additional body cooling. *Electroencephalogr. Clin. Neurophysiol.* **1985**, *60*, 33–38. [CrossRef] [PubMed]
41. Kräuchi, K.; Cajochen, C.; Werth, E.; Wirz-Justice, A. Warm feet promote the rapid onset of sleep. *Nature* **1999**, *401*, 36–37. [CrossRef] [PubMed]
42. Murphy, P.J.; Campbell, S.S. Nighttime drop in body temperature: A physiological trigger for sleep onset? *Sleep* **1997**, *20*, 505–511. [CrossRef] [PubMed]
43. Uchida, S.; Shioda, K.; Morita, Y.; Kubota, C.; Ganeko, M.; Takeda, N. Exercise effects on sleep physiology. *Front. Neurol.* **2012**, *3*, 48. [CrossRef] [PubMed]
44. Taheri, M.; Irandoust, K. The exercise-induced weight loss improves self-reported quality of sleep in obese elderly women with sleep disorders. *Sleep Hypn.* **2018**, *20*, 54–59. [CrossRef]
45. Morres, I.D.; Hatzigeorgiadis, A.; Stathi, A.; Comoutos, N.; Arpin-Cribbie, C.; Krommidas, C.; Theodorakis, Y. Aerobic exercise for adult patients with major depressive disorder in mental health services: A systematic review and meta-analysis. *Depress. Anxiety* **2019**, *36*, 39–53. [CrossRef]
46. Aylett, E.; Small, N.; Bower, P. Exercise in the treatment of clinical anxiety in general practice—A systematic review and meta-analysis. *BMC Health Serv. Res.* **2018**, *18*, 559. [CrossRef]
47. Björkman, F.; Ekblom, Ö. Physical exercise as treatment for PTSD: A systematic review and meta-analysis. *Mil. Med.* **2022**, *187*, e1103–e1113. [CrossRef]
48. Vancampfort, D.; Hallgren, M.; Firth, J.; Rosenbaum, S.; Schuch, F.B.; Mugisha, J.; Probst, M.; Van Damme, T.; Carvalho, A.F.; Stubbs, B. Physical activity and suicidal ideation: A systematic review and meta-analysis. *J. Affect. Disord.* **2018**, *225*, 438–448. [CrossRef]

Disclaimer/Publisher's Note: The statements, opinions and data contained in all publications are solely those of the individual author(s) and contributor(s) and not of MDPI and/or the editor(s). MDPI and/or the editor(s) disclaim responsibility for any injury to people or property resulting from any ideas, methods, instructions or products referred to in the content.

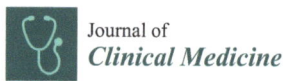

Article

The Interplay of Sleep Quality, Mental Health, and Sociodemographic and Clinical Factors among Italian College Freshmen

Jessica Dagani [1], Chiara Buizza [1], Herald Cela [2], Giulio Sbravati [1], Giuseppe Rainieri [1] and Alberto Ghilardi [1,*]

[1] Department of Clinical and Experimental Sciences, University of Brescia, Viale Europa 11, 25123 Brescia, Italy; j.dagani@studenti.unibs.it (J.D.); chiara.buizza@unibs.it (C.B.); giulio.sbravati@unibs.it (G.S.); giuseppe.rainieri@unibs.it (G.R.)
[2] Department of Psychology, University of Graz, Universitätsplatz 2, 8010 Graz, Austria
* Correspondence: alberto.ghilardi@unibs.it

Abstract: Background/Objectives: Sleep and mental health are closely linked, with sleep deprivation increasing the risk of mental health problems in college students. This study aimed to analyze the role of sleep in the mental health status of a sample of Italian freshmen, considering various mental health outcomes and potential interactions between sleep and other relevant factors, such as sociodemographic characteristics, academic experiences, and mental health history. **Methods**: All freshmen from a medium-sized Italian university were invited to participate in a multidimensional online survey (n = 3756). Sleep quality was assessed through questions on average hours of sleep per night and on satisfaction of perceived sleep quality. Mental health outcomes included psychophysical well-being, psychological distress, substance use, and problematic internet use. Statistical analysis involved multivariate analysis of variance, followed by pairwise comparisons. **Results**: The sample (n = 721) exhibited low levels of well-being and a high prevalence of psychological distress (52.1%). Approximately one-third of students (n = 258) were dissatisfied with their sleep quality, and one-fourth (n = 186) reported inadequate sleep (less than 7 h per night). More specifically, 24.4% of students slept on average six hours per night, and 1.4% slept five hours or less. Satisfaction with perceived sleep quality significantly influenced well-being, psychological distress, and cannabis use (η_p^2 = 0.02). Interaction effects were observed between satisfaction with sleep quality and drop-out intentions (η_p^2 = 0.01), as well as between satisfaction with sleep quality and history of mental health diagnosis (η_p^2 = 0.02), both of which were significant for psychological distress and cannabis use. **Conclusions**: This study highlights the influence of perceived sleep quality on academic distress among college freshmen, particularly those with higher intentions of leaving university and with a history of mental health diagnosis.

Keywords: sleep; college freshmen; mental health; well-being; psychological distress

1. Introduction

Mental health issues are prevalent among university students, with the academic environment introducing various stressors, such as increased workload and lifestyle adjustments, including changes in sleep and eating habits [1,2]. Indeed, poor sleep hygiene is prevalent among college students, characterized by insufficient sleep duration and low sleep quality [3,4]. This might be particularly pronounced among freshmen, who are often more vulnerable to the challenges of adapting to the new stressful academic environment [5,6]. A recent European cross-sectional study found support for this, showing a higher prevalence of insomnia symptoms among newer university students [7].

Students' mental health is influenced by a myriad of factors, including sociodemographic characteristics, mental health history, academic experience, and lifestyle habits. For instance, gender and relationship status have been associated with stress levels among

Australian nursing students [8], while students with a family or personal history of mental illness are at higher risk of developing mental health problems in university [9]. Moreover, students who opt to leave university often grapple with mental health challenges [10]. Research also indicates a correlation between mental health symptoms and poor sleep [3,11], with sleep problems in college students having serious consequences, including cognitive deficits, risky behaviors, impaired relationships, and overall poor health [12,13]. Two large-scale studies involving American college students found significant associations between anxiety and depression symptoms with poor sleep quality [14,15]. Additionally, a meta-analysis by Scott and colleagues [16] on sleep-improvement interventions suggested a causal relationship between sleep and mental health difficulties. Moreover, insomnia has been linked to decreased academic performance and unhealthy behaviors [4,17], which are highly prevalent among university students, including problematic internet use and alcohol/cannabis misuse [18–20]. While research on problematic internet use and its associations with sleep has primarily focused on adolescents [21,22], some studies on university students have reported similar significant associations [23,24]. Concerning alcohol consumption, evidence suggests that it may exacerbate sleep problems [25], although findings from university student cohorts are not entirely consistent [6,11]. Similarly, hazardous cannabis use has been linked to insomnia symptoms among college students [26,27], but further research is needed to better understand the nature of this association.

The aim of the present study was to explore the role of sleep in the mental health status of a large sample of Italian freshmen, considering various mental health outcomes and potential interactions with sleep and sociodemographic characteristics, health history, and academic factors.

2. Materials and Methods

2.1. Study Design

This cross-sectional observational study involved freshmen from a medium-sized university in northern Italy. Data collection took place from May to June 2022. In collaboration with the University administration, an email invitation was sent to all freshmen enrolled in the academic year 2021/2022 to participate in a multidimensional online survey created with LimeSurvey (www.limesurvey.org), a tool ensuring completely anonymous data collection. The email included a description of the study and a link to access the survey. Upon accessing the web link, participants were asked to provide informed consent before proceeding with the survey. LimeSurvey automatically removed any participant identifiers from the survey data, delivering only deidentified data to the investigators. Organizational ethics approval was obtained from the Board of Directors of the University of Brescia (approved with provision no. 330 on 22 November 2021). The survey was conducted in accordance with the World Medical Association's Helsinki Declaration for Human Studies.

2.2. Survey Instrument

This multidimensional survey assessed a wide range of sociodemographic and academic characteristics, as well as multiple aspects related to students' psychological and physical well-being. Sleep quality was assessed through two questions: a question about the average number of hours slept per night and another on the satisfaction with perceived sleep quality. More specifically, students were asked the following open-ended question: "How many hours of sleep do you get per night on average?" and were asked to estimate their usual sleep duration to the nearest whole hour. The number of hours slept per night was further dichotomized into two categories: "less than seven hours" and "seven or more hours". Satisfaction with perceived sleep quality was measured on a five-point Likert scale ranging from 0 ("Very dissatisfied") to 4 ("Very satisfied"), with participants later classified into three categories based on their answers: Dissatisfied (0 = "Very dissatisfied" or 1 = "Quite dissatisfied"), Neither satisfied nor dissatisfied (2 = "Neither satisfied nor dissatisfied"), and Satisfied (3 = "Quite dissatisfied" or 4 = "Very dissatisfied"). In our analyses, we primarily focused on two of these categories: the Dissatisfied students and the

Satisfied students. We specifically focused on students who clearly and distinctly expressed either satisfaction or dissatisfaction with their quality of sleep (as opposed to those who appeared neutral) in order to more precisely assess the impact of this satisfaction on mental health outcomes.

To evaluate students' mental health status, we included measures of psychophysical well-being and psychological distress related to academic stressors as outcome measures. We opted for psychophysical well-being as it encompasses a broad range of emotional and psychological experiences of college students, and we included psychological distress related to academic stressors as a construct specific to our sample, given the constant pressures of academic demands experienced by college students [28]. Additionally, we incorporated measures related to prevalent unhealthy behaviors among students, such as problematic internet use and the use of alcohol and cannabis. The inclusion of these measures provided a more comprehensive approach to mental health status, considering their high prevalence among students and their impact on several mental health aspects [23,29–32].

More specifically, the survey included the following standardized tools:

- General Health Questionnaire (GHQ-12) [33]. The GHQ-12 is a widely used self-administered rating scale assessing mental health and psychophysical well-being. It comprises 12 questions with a four-point response scale. In this study, we used the standard bimodal method (0-0-1-1) of scoring, where a score of 0 is assigned to the first two low-stress alternatives and a score of 1 is given to the two high-stress alternatives. Total scores range from 0 to 12, with scores above 3 indicating psychological distress. The GHQ-12 showed good reliability in our sample, as indicated by a Cronbach's alpha value of 0.78.
- University Stress Scale (USS) [34]. The USS is a 21-item screening test measuring the cognitive appraisal of demands across the range of environmental stressors experienced by students. Each item is rated on a four-point Likert scale (0 = "Not at all", 3 = "Constantly"). The sum of all items gives the extent score, ranging from 0 to 63. An extent score of 13 or higher indicates significant psychological distress. The USS showed high reliability in our sample, as measured by a Cronbach's alpha value of 0.85.
- A modified version of World Health Organization-ASSIST v3.0 (ASSIST). The ASSIST is a questionnaire aimed at evaluating substance use for ten different substances: tobacco, alcohol, cannabis, cocaine, amphetamine-type stimulants, inhalants, sedatives, hallucinogens, opioids, and "other drugs". A score is determined for each substance and categorized as low (occasional or nonharmful use), moderate (more regular use or harmful/hazardous use), or high-risk use (frequent high-risk use or suggestive of dependence). In this study, we employed the self-report adaptation of Barreto and colleagues [35] and focused on alcohol and cannabis use patterns, due to their prevalence among students. Participants were categorized as low-risk or moderate/high-risk users based on established cut-off scores (10 for alcohol and 3 for cannabis). The ASSIST's ability to classify drug use severity has been extensively validated [36,37]. In our sample, Cronbach's alpha values were confirmed at 0.56 for alcohol and at 0.79 for cannabis.
- Internet Abusive Use Questionnaire (IAUQ) [38]. The IAUQ assesses problematic internet use and includes 12 items rated on a five-point Likert scale (0 = "totally disagree", 4 = "totally agree"). The total score ranges from 0 to 48 and the author suggested a cut-off of 24 as indicative of problematic internet use. We categorized participants based on their total score: nonproblematic internet use (below the cut-off) and problematic internet use (above the cut-off). In this sample, the IAUQ demonstrated high reliability, as measured by a Cronbach's alpha value of 0.90.

2.3. Data Analysis

This study aimed to explore the relationship between sleep patterns and mental health outcomes among college students. The analysis included correlation analysis, multivariate analysis of variance (MANOVA), and follow-up univariate analyses (ANOVAs) with pairwise comparisons.

Descriptive statistics were computed for sociodemographic and clinical characteristics, as well as for questionnaire scores. Categorical variables were summarized using percentage distributions, while means and standard deviations (SD) were used for quantitative variables.

Prior to MANOVA, correlations among the dependent variables were examined to assess multicollinearity. Pearson correlation coefficients were calculated between the mental health measures (outcome variables), including USS, GHQ-12, ASSIST for alcohol and cannabis use, and IAUQ.

A MANOVA was performed to assess the overall differences in mental health outcomes across groups defined by the predictors, including sleep patterns (perceived sleep quality and average hours of sleep per night) and demographic factors (gender, employment status, relationship status, field of study, drop-out intentions, lifetime psychological support, and lifetime mental health diagnosis). Pillai's Trace was chosen among the multivariate tests due to its conservative nature and robustness to violations of assumptions.

Significant results from the MANOVA were followed up with univariate analyses (ANOVAs) to examine the effects of individual predictors on each mental health outcome separately. Bonferroni correction was applied to adjust for multiple comparisons when conducting pairwise comparisons between groups.

Pairwise comparisons were conducted using estimated marginal means to examine differences between specific groups or levels of the predictors. Bonferroni correction was applied to control the family-wise error rate in the pairwise comparisons.

All statistical analyses were conducted using IBM SPSS Statistics (version 29). The significance level was set at $\alpha = 0.05$ for all tests.

3. Results
3.1. Characteristics of the Sample

Among the 3756 freshmen in the study population, 721 (19.2%) completed the survey. The participants had a mean age of 20.83 years (SD = 3.83), and the majority (63.4%) were female. Most students (70.6%) had never received psychological support, and only 6.1% had ever received a diagnosis of a mental disorder. Notably, a high proportion of students (81.3%) scored above the cut-off point on the GHQ-12, indicating low levels of psychophysical well-being. Similarly, over half of the participants (52.1%) scored in the range indicating significant psychological distress on the USS. Regarding sleep patterns, 24.4% of students indicated sleeping an average of six hours per night, while only a limited number (1.4%) indicated sleeping five hours or less. Conversely, only three participants reported sleeping more than nine hours per night. Additional sample characteristics are reported in Table 1.

3.2. Multivariate Analysis

Statistical analysis showed significant correlations between the dependent variables (Pearson coefficients for significant correlations ranging from 0.089 to 0.423; see Supplementary Materials Table S1), supporting the rationale for conducting a MANOVA to further explore the relationships and differences across groups defined by the predictors. Table 2 displays significant multivariate effects observed for predictors included in the analysis, such as gender, satisfaction with perceived quality of sleep, lifetime psychological support, lifetime diagnosis of mental disorder, and drop-out intentions. In addition, significant effects were detected also for the interactions of sleep satisfaction both with drop-out intentions and with the lifetime diagnosis of a mental disorder.

Univariates with post hoc analysis revealed significant differences among students reporting different levels of sleep satisfaction in GHQ-12 total score ($F(2, 672) = 3.79$, $p = 0.023$, $\eta_p^2 = 0.01$), USS total score ($F(2, 672) = 3.92$, $p = 0.020$, $\eta_p^2 = 0.01$), and ASSIST Cannabis total score ($F(2, 672) = 8.65$, $p < 0.001$, $\eta_p^2 = 0.02$). Specifically, students dissatisfied with their sleep quality showed a higher GHQ-12 total score compared with students neither satisfied nor dissatisfied (mean difference = 3.92 points, SE = 1.25, $p = 0.026$, 95% CI [0.29, 6.29]). Moreover, students dissatisfied with their sleep quality exhibited significantly higher USS total scores compared with satisfied students (mean difference = 4.20 points, SE = 1.68, $p = 0.039$, 95% CI [0.16, 8.24]). In addition, students dissatisfied with their sleep quality demonstrated significantly higher ASSIST Cannabis total scores compared with both satisfied students (mean difference = 2.196 points, SE = 0.73, $p = 0.008$, 95% CI [0.45, 3.94]) and neither satisfied nor dissatisfied students (mean difference = 2.799 points, SE = 0.709, $p < 0.001$, 95% CI [1.10, 4.50]).

Table 1. Characteristics of the sample.

Variable	n	%
Relationship Status		
Single	405	56.2
With a partner	314	43.6
Missing	2	0.2
Employment status		
Student	473	65.6
Student worker	248	34.4
Field of Study		
Medicine and Pharmacy	325	45.1
Engineering and Agricultural	170	23.6
Economics	180	25.0
Law	46	6.4
Satisfaction with perceived quality of sleep		
Dissatisfied	258	35.8
Neither satisfied nor dissatisfied	170	23.6
Satisfied	293	40.6
Hours of sleep per night		
Less than 7 h	186	25.8
Equal or more than 7 h	532	73.8
Missing	3	0.4
ASSIST—Level of risky use of alcohol		
Low risk	638	88.5
Medium/high risk	83	11.5
ASSIST—Level of risky use of cannabis		
Low risk	670	92.9
Medium/high risk	51	7.1
Intentions to drop out of university		
Low intentions	514	71.3
Medium/high intentions	207	28.7
	Mean	SD
Hours of sleep per night	7.02	1.04
GHQ-12 total score	6.07	2.91
USS total score	14.43	8.39
IAUQ total score	12.43	9.43
ASSIST Alcohol Total Score	4.71	5.04
ASSIST Cannabis Total Score	0.84	3.33

3.3. Interactions among Perceived Sleep Quality and Other Factors

In exploring interactions with pairwise comparisons, we report here only significant differences between students dissatisfied versus students satisfied with their sleep quality. For the other comparisons, refer to Supplementary Materials (Table S2).

The interaction between satisfaction with perceived sleep quality and drop-out intentions showed significant differences in USS total score ($F(2, 672) = 8.29$, $p < 0.001$, $\eta_p^2 = 0.02$). Specifically, among students with medium/high intentions to drop out, those dissatisfied with their sleep quality had a mean USS total score that was 7.51 points higher compared with those satisfied with their sleep quality (SE = 1.98, $p < 0.001$, 95% CI [2.76, 12.27]).

Table 2. Multivariate analysis.

Effect	Pillai's Trace	F	df$_{num}$	df$_{den}$	p	η_p^2
Gender	0.053	7.485	5.000	668.000	<0.001	0.053
Relationship status	0.002	0.223	5.000	668.000	0.953	0.002
Field of study	0.035	1.595	15.000	2010.000	0.067	0.012
Employment status	0.009	1.270	5.000	668.000	0.275	0.009
Sleep satisfaction	0.043	2.957	10.000	1338.000	0.001	0.022
Hours of sleep	0.003	0.377	5.000	668.000	0.865	0.003
Psychological support lifetime	0.017	2.280	5.000	668.000	0.045	0.017
Diagnosis of mental disorder lifetime	0.020	2.703	5.000	668.000	0.020	0.020
Drop-out intentions	0.084	12.225	5.000	668.000	<0.001	0.084
Gender × Sleep satisfaction	0.018	1.238	10.000	1338.000	0.262	0.009
Relationship status × Sleep satisfaction	0.016	1.048	10.000	1338.000	0.400	0.008
Field of study × Sleep satisfaction	0.053	1.193	30.000	3360.000	0.217	0.011
Employment status × Sleep satisfaction	0.026	1.781	10.000	1338.000	0.059	0.013
Psychological support lifetime × Sleep satisfaction	0.005	0.360	10.000	1338.000	0.963	0.003
Diagnosis of mental disorder lifetime × Sleep satisfaction	0.040	2.744	10.000	1338.000	0.002	0.020
Drop-out intentions × Sleep satisfaction	0.029	1.978	10.000	1338.000	0.032	0.015
Gender × Hours of sleep	0.014	1.953	5.000	668.000	0.084	0.014
Relationship status × Hours of sleep	0.009	1.187	5.000	668.000	0.314	0.009
Field of study × Hours of sleep	0.035	1.582	15.000	2010.000	0.071	0.012
Employment status × Hours of sleep	0.002	0.276	5.000	668.000	0.927	0.002
Psychological support lifetime × Hours of sleep	0.006	0.848	5.000	668.000	0.516	0.006
Diagnosis of mental disorder lifetime × Hours of sleep	0.001	0.168	5.000	668.000	0.974	0.001
Drop-out intentions × Hours of sleep	0.003	0.366	5.000	668.000	0.872	0.003

Multivariate analysis with Pillai's Trace on collected variables, analyzing both main effects and interactions for sleep variables. η_p^2 = partial eta squared.

The interaction between satisfaction with perceived sleep quality and lifetime mental health diagnosis showed significant differences in ASSIST Cannabis total score (F(2, 672) = 7.56, $p < 0.001$, $\eta_p^2 = 0.02$). Specifically, among students who have had a diagnosis of a mental disorder, those dissatisfied with their sleep quality had a mean ASSIST Cannabis total score that was 4.48 points higher compared with those satisfied with their sleep quality (SE = 1.35, $p = 0.003$, 95% CI [1.23, 7.73]).

4. Discussion

This study aimed to explore the aggregate effect of sleep on various mental health outcomes among college freshmen, both independently and in interaction with other variables. Results from descriptive analysis supported previous findings on the poor mental health status of college students [39–41] and confirmed the prevalence of sleep problems previously highlighted in similar samples [3,4]. Considering sleep duration guidelines which recommend at least seven hours per night for young adults [42], one in four students in our sample did not get enough sleep and about one in three was not satisfied with their sleep quality. Our results contrast with those of previous Italian and European studies, where approximately half (or more) of students reported insufficient sleep quality [43–45]. This discrepancy may be attributed to methodological differences, as those studies employed standardized sleep assessment tools while our study relied on self-reported sleep measures.

Furthermore, the main results show that, among other factors, perceived sleep quality was associated with mental health outcomes, consistent with previous research [14,46,47]. Sleep and mental health are closely intertwined, with sleep deprivation increasing the risk of developing mental health problems, which can then detrimentally impact academic performance [48]. Perceived sleep quality specifically influences measures of psychological distress and cannabis use, even when considering its interactions with drop-out intentions and a history of mental disorder diagnosis. Regarding drop-out intentions, results reveal that among students with medium/high intentions of leaving university, perceived sleep quality was significantly and substantially associated with perceived academic distress. This suggests that feeling well-rested might be particularly crucial for students already contemplating leaving university. The stress of a major decision, coupled with fatigue from poor sleep, may exacerbate existing academic pressures and significantly increase their distress levels.

Perceived sleep quality, when considered alongside a lifetime diagnosis of a mental disorder, appeared to correlate with differences in cannabis consumption, as students dissatisfied with their sleep quality tended to report significantly higher scores. Given the increased vulnerability of students with a history of mental disorders to experiencing mental health problems in university [9], it is plausible that poor sleep quality could potentially contribute to some students' decision to self-medicate in an attempt to improve sleep [49]. However, it is important to note that while low perceived sleep quality and resulting discomfort may suggest a link to cannabis self-medication to alleviate distress [50], further research is needed to confirm this hypothesis.

This study suggests a strong connection between sleep habits, substance use, and mental health in college students. Healthy sleep habits might be particularly important for students at risk of dropping out or using substances, as sleep problems and resulting distress may lead them to seek coping mechanisms like substance use [51]. Additionally, healthy sleep habits have the potential to be particularly beneficial for vulnerable students, such as those already diagnosed with a mental disorder, where substance use may further deteriorate their mental health [50].

While our study focused on examining the relationship between sleep and mental health outcomes among college freshmen, it is crucial to acknowledge the broader context of student well-being. Promoting good sleep could be an important component of a broader program aimed at improving student well-being. The university lifestyle can foster unhealthy behaviors like lack of exercise, which can further impact sleep quality and overall health [52]. Adequate sleep plays a crucial role in managing stress, which is a common challenge among college students due to academic, social, and extracurricular commitments [53]. Quality sleep can help reduce stress, improve coping skills, and enhance academic performance, potentially due to better memory, concentration, and problem-solving abilities [48,54,55].

While our study sheds light on the relationship between sleep and mental health outcomes among college freshmen, future research should continue to explore these relationships to develop more effective interventions and support mechanisms for promoting student well-being. Universities might consider strengthening their counseling services to provide adequate support for students struggling with stress and sleep issues. Promoting a culture of well-being can not only benefit students' personal health and future prospects but also have significant positive implications from social and economic perspectives.

Limitations

This study has some limitations, mainly concerning the generalizability of the results. Data were gathered only from freshmen at a single university in northern Italy, and voluntary participation may have introduced selection bias, as students who participated might differ from those who declined. Further studies including more representative samples and cross-cultural comparisons are therefore needed. The self-report nature of our assessments is a second limitation, potentially affecting the validity of the results. Additionally, while we used two measures to assess sleep (number of hours and perceived quality), employing a more comprehensive and standardized questionnaire would have allowed for a more accurate and detailed assessment, facilitating comparisons with other studies. Another limitation is that we focused on specific mental health outcomes, such as psychophysical well-being, university distress, substance use, and problematic internet use.

These chosen outcomes, while providing a broad view of the emotional and psychological experiences of college students, may not capture the full spectrum of their mental health. Furthermore, the results regarding cannabis use should be interpreted with caution due to the low number of students using this substance and their reporting of medium/high-risk use. Social desirability bias might also have led to an underestimation of actual use.

5. Conclusions

This study contributes to understanding the role of sleep in the mental health of college freshmen by examining various mental health outcomes and interactions with sociodemographic and clinical factors. Our findings revealed a high prevalence of poor sleep quality and dissatisfaction among students. Notably, perceived sleep quality showed a strong association with psychological distress, particularly among those considering dropping out. Furthermore, among freshmen with the highest drop-out intentions, those reporting the most dissatisfaction with sleep quality also reported the highest cannabis use. These findings highlight the potential value of exploring interventions aimed at enhancing sleep quality and promoting healthy lifestyle choices among college students. Further research is warranted to gain a deeper understanding of the complex interaction that exists between sleep, mental health, and other sociodemographic, clinical, and academic factors.

Supplementary Materials: The following supporting information can be downloaded at https://www.mdpi.com/article/10.3390/jcm13092626/s1, Table S1: Correlations between outcome variables; Table S2. Pairwise correlations satisfaction with sleep quality.

Author Contributions: J.D. contributed to data analysis and interpretation and wrote a first draft of the paper. C.B. and A.G. conceptualized the idea of the paper, supervised the study, and contributed to writing the first draft of the paper. G.S. and G.R. carried out the web surveys and data collection. H.C. conducted data analysis and contributed to data interpretation and manuscript revision. All authors have read and agreed to the published version of the manuscript.

Funding: This work received a specific grant from the Italian Ministry of University and Research for tutoring orientation actions, as well as recovery and inclusion actions, also with reference to students with disabilities and specific learning disabilities (D.M. n. 752, 30 June 2021).

Institutional Review Board Statement: This study was conducted in accordance with the Declaration of Helsinki and approved by the Institutional Review Board of Directors of the University of Brescia (approved with provision no. 330 on 22 November 2021).

Informed Consent Statement: Informed consent was obtained from all subjects involved in this study.

Data Availability Statement: The data that support the findings of this study are available upon request from the corresponding author.

Conflicts of Interest: The authors declare no conflicts of interest.

References

1. Bruffaerts, R.; Mortier, P.; Auerbach, R.P.; Alonso, J.; De la Torre, A.E.H.; Cuijpers, P.; Demyttenaere, K.; Ebert, D.D.; Green, J.G.; Hasking, P.; et al. Lifetime and 12-Month Treatment for Mental Disorders and Suicidal Thoughts and Behaviors among First-Year College Students. *Int. J. Methods Psychiatr. Res.* **2019**, *28*, e1764. [CrossRef] [PubMed]
2. Saleh, D.; Camart, N.; Romo, L. Predictors of Stress in College Students. *Front. Psychol.* **2017**, *8*, 19. [CrossRef] [PubMed]
3. Gardani, M.; Bradford, D.R.R.; Russell, K.; Allan, S.; Beattie, L.; Ellis, J.G.; Akram, U. A Systematic Review and Meta-Analysis of Poor Sleep, Insomnia Symptoms and Stress in Undergraduate Students. *Sleep Med. Rev.* **2022**, *61*, 101565. [CrossRef]
4. Seoane, H.A.; Moschetto, L.; Orliacq, F.; Orliacq, J.; Serrano, E.; Cazenave, M.I.; Vigo, D.E.; Perez-Lloret, S. Sleep Disruption in Medicine Students and Its Relationship with Impaired Academic Performance: A Systematic Review and Meta-Analysis. *Sleep Med. Rev.* **2020**, *53*, 101333. [CrossRef] [PubMed]
5. Cheng, S.H.; Shih, C.C.; Lee, I.H.; Hou, Y.W.; Chen, K.C.; Chen, K.T.; Yang, Y.K.; Yang, Y.C. A Study on the Sleep Quality of Incoming University Students. *Psychiatry Res.* **2012**, *197*, 270–274. [CrossRef] [PubMed]
6. Li, Y.; Bai, W.; Zhu, B.; Duan, R.; Yu, X.; Xu, W.; Wang, M.; Hua, W.; Yu, W.; Li, W.; et al. Prevalence and Correlates of Poor Sleep Quality Among College Students: A Cross-Sectional Survey. *Health Qual. Life Outcomes* **2020**, *18*, 210. [CrossRef] [PubMed]
7. Navarro-Martínez, R.; Chover-Sierra, E.; Colomer-Pérez, N.; Vlachou, E.; Andriuseviciene, V.; Cauli, O. Sleep Quality and Its Association with Substance Abuse Among University Students. *Clin. Neurol. Neurosurg.* **2020**, *188*, 105591. [CrossRef] [PubMed]

8. Asturias, N.; Andrew, S.; Boardman, G.; Kerr, D. The Influence of Socio-Demographic Factors on Stress and Coping Strategies among Undergraduate Nursing Students. *Nurse Educ. Today* **2021**, *99*, 104780. [CrossRef]
9. Campbell, F.; Blank, L.; Cantrell, A.; Baxter, S.; Blackmore, C.; Dixon, J.; Goyder, E. Factors that Influence Mental Health of University and College Students in the UK: A Systematic Review. *BMC Public Health* **2022**, *22*, 1778. [CrossRef]
10. Hjorth, C.F.; Bilgrav, L.; Frandsen, L.S.; Overgaard, C.; Torp-Pedersen, C.; Nielsen, B.; Bøggild, H. Mental Health and School Drop-Out Across Educational Levels and Genders: A 4.8-Year Follow-Up Study. *BMC Public Health* **2016**, *16*, 976. [CrossRef]
11. Lund, H.G.; Reider, B.D.; Whiting, A.B.; Prichard, J.R. Sleep Patterns and Predictors of Disturbed Sleep in a Large Population of College Students. *J. Adolesc. Health* **2010**, *46*, 124–132. [CrossRef] [PubMed]
12. Carney, C.E.; Edinger, J.D.; Meyer, B. Daily Activities and Sleep Quality in College Students. *Chronobiol Int.* **2006**, *23*, 623–637 [CrossRef] [PubMed]
13. O'Brien, E.M.; Mindell, J.A. Sleep and Risk-Taking Behavior in Adolescents. *Behav. Sleep Med.* **2005**, *3*, 113–133. [CrossRef] [PubMed]
14. Becker, S.P.; Jarrett, M.A.; Luebbe, A.M.; Garner, A.A.; Burns, G.L.; Kofler, M.J. Sleep in a Large, Multi-University Sample of College Students: Sleep Problem Prevalence, Sex Differences, and Mental Health Correlates. *Sleep Health* **2018**, *4*, 174–181 [CrossRef] [PubMed]
15. Boehm, M.A.; Lei, Q.M.; Lloyd, R.M.; Prichard, J.R. Depression, Anxiety, and Tobacco Use: Overlapping Impediments to Sleep in a National Sample of College Students. *J. Am. Coll. Health* **2016**, *64*, 565–574. [CrossRef] [PubMed]
16. Scott, A.J.; Webb, T.L.; Martyn-St James, M.; Rowse, G.; Weich, S. Improving Sleep Quality Leads to Better Mental Health: A Meta-Analysis of Randomized Controlled Trials. *Sleep Med. Rev.* **2021**, *60*, 101556. [CrossRef] [PubMed]
17. Carrión-Pantoja, S.; Prados, G.; Chouchou, F.; Holguín, M.; Mendoza-Vinces, Á.; Expósito-Ruiz, M.; Fernández-Puerta, L. Insomnia Symptoms, Sleep Hygiene, Mental Health, and Academic Performance in Spanish University Students: A Cross Sectional Study. *J. Clin. Med.* **2022**, *11*, 1989. [CrossRef] [PubMed]
18. Schulenberg, J.E.; Johnston, L.D.; O'Malley, P.M.; Bachman, J.G.; Miech, R.A.; Patrick, M.E. *Monitoring the Future National Survey Results on Drug Use, 1975–2018: Volume II, College Students and Adults Ages 19–60*; Institute for Social Research, The University of Michigan: Ann Arbor, MI, USA, 2019.
19. Stevens, C.; Zhang, E.; Cherkerzian, S.; Chen, J.A.; Liu, C.H. Problematic Internet Use/Computer Gaming Among US College Students: Prevalence and Correlates with Mental Health Symptoms. *Depress. Anxiety* **2020**, *37*, 1127–1136. [CrossRef] [PubMed]
20. Wang, Q.; Liu, Y.; Wang, B.; An, Y.; Wang, H.; Zhang, Y.; Mati, K. Problematic Internet Use and Subjective Sleep Quality Among College Students in China: Results from a Pilot Study. *J. Am. Coll. Health* **2022**, *70*, 552–560. [CrossRef]
21. de Sá, S.; Baião, A.; Marques, H.; Marques, M.D.C.; Reis, M.J.; Dias, S.; Catarino, M. The Influence of Smartphones on Adolescent Sleep: A Systematic Literature Review. *Nurs. Rep.* **2023**, *13*, 612–621. [CrossRef]
22. Kokka, I.; Mourikis, I.; Nicolaides, N.C.; Darviri, C.; Chrousos, G.P.; Kanaka-Gantenbein, C.; Bacopoulou, F. Exploring the Effects of Problematic Internet Use on Adolescent Sleep: A Systematic Review. *Int. J. Environ. Res. Public Health* **2021**, *18*, 760. [CrossRef] [PubMed]
23. Demirci, K.; Akgönül, M.; Akpinar, A. Relationship of Smartphone Use Severity with Sleep Quality, Depression, and Anxiety in University Students. *J. Behav. Addict.* **2015**, *4*, 85–92. [CrossRef] [PubMed]
24. Rathakrishnan, B.; Bikar Singh, S.S.; Kamaluddin, M.R.; Yahaya, A.; Mohd Nasir, M.A.; Ibrahim, F.; Ab Rahman, Z. Smartphone Addiction and Sleep Quality on Academic Performance of University Students: An Exploratory Research. *Int. J. Environ. Res Public Health* **2021**, *18*, 8291. [CrossRef]
25. Hu, N.; Ma, Y.; He, J.; Zhu, L.; Cao, S. Alcohol Consumption and Incidence of Sleep Disorder: A Systematic Review and Meta-Analysis of Cohort Studies. *Drug Alcohol Depend.* **2020**, *217*, 108259. [CrossRef]
26. Keen, L., 2nd; Turner, A.D.; George, L.; Lawrence, K. Cannabis Use Disorder Severity and Sleep Quality Among Undergraduates Attending a Historically Black University. *Addict. Behav.* **2022**, *134*, 107414. [CrossRef]
27. Wong, M.M.; Craun, E.A.; Bravo, A.J.; Pearson, M.R.; Protective Strategies Study Team. Insomnia Symptoms, Cannabis Protective Behavioral Strategies, and Hazardous Cannabis Use Among U.S. College Students. *Exp. Clin. Psychopharmacol.* **2019**, *27*, 309–317 [CrossRef] [PubMed]
28. Baik, C.; Larcombe, W.; Brooker, A. How Universities Can Enhance Student Mental Well-Being: The Student Perspective. *High Educ. Res. Dev.* **2019**, *38*, 674–687. [CrossRef]
29. Cai, Z.; Mao, P.; Wang, Z.; Wang, D.; He, J.; Fan, X. Associations between Problematic Internet Use and Mental Health Outcomes of Students: A Meta-Analytic Review. *Adolesc. Res. Rev.* **2023**, *8*, 45–62. [CrossRef] [PubMed]
30. Hall, W.D. Cannabis Use and the Mental Health of Young People. *Aust. N. Z. J. Psychiatry* **2006**, *40*, 105–113. [CrossRef]
31. Sæther, S.M.M.; Knapstad, M.; Askeland, K.G.; Skogen, J.C. Alcohol Consumption, Life Satisfaction and Mental Health Among Norwegian College and University Students. *Addict. Behav. Rep.* **2019**, *10*, 100216. [CrossRef]
32. Tembo, C.; Burns, S.; Kalembo, F. The Association between Levels of Alcohol Consumption and Mental Health Problems and Academic Performance Among Young University Students. *PLoS ONE* **2017**, *12*, e0178142. [CrossRef] [PubMed]
33. Goldberg, D.P.; Blackwell, B. Psychiatric Illness in General Practice: A Detailed Study Using a New Method of Case Identification *Br. Med. J.* **1970**, *1*, 439–443. [CrossRef] [PubMed]
34. Stallman, H.; Hurst, C. The University Stress Scale: Measuring Domains and Extent of Stress in University Students. *Austral Psychol.* **2016**, *51*, 128–134. [CrossRef]

35. Barreto, H.A.; de Oliveira Christoff, A.; Boerngen-Lacerda, R. Development of a Self-Report Format of ASSIST with University Students. *Addict. Behav.* **2014**, *39*, 1152–1158. [CrossRef] [PubMed]
36. Humeniuk, R.; Ali, R.; Babor, T.F.; Farrell, M.; Formigoni, M.L.; Jittiwutikarn, J.; de Lacerda, R.B.; Ling, W.; Marsden, J.; Monteiro, M.; et al. Validation of the Alcohol, Smoking and Substance Involvement Screening Test (ASSIST). *Addiction* **2008**, *103*, 1039–1047. [CrossRef] [PubMed]
37. Humeniuk, R.; Ali, R.; Babor, T.; Souza-Formigoni, M.L.O.; de Lacerda, R.B.; Ling, W.; McRee, B.; Newcombe, D.; Pal, H.; Poznyak, V.; et al. A Randomized Controlled Trial of a Brief Intervention for Illicit Drugs Linked to the Alcohol, Smoking and Substance Involvement Screening Test (ASSIST) in Clients Recruited from Primary Health-Care Settings in Four Countries. *Addiction* **2012**, *107*, 957–966. [CrossRef]
38. Calvo-Francés, F. Internet Abusive Use Questionnaire: Psychometric Properties. *Comput. Hum. Behav.* **2016**, *59*, 187–194. [CrossRef]
39. Al-Khani, A.M.; Sarhandi, M.I.; Zaghloul, M.S.; Ewid, M.; Saquib, N. A Cross-Sectional Survey on Sleep Quality, Mental Health, and Academic Performance among Medical Students in Saudi Arabia. *BMC Res. Notes* **2019**, *12*, 665. [CrossRef]
40. Auerbach, R.P.; Mortier, P.; Bruffaerts, R.; Alonso, J.; Benjet, C.; Cuijpers, P.; Demyttenaere, K.; Ebert, D.D.; Green, J.G.; Hasking, P.; et al. WHO World Mental Health Surveys International College Student Project: Prevalence and Distribution of Mental Disorders. *J. Abnorm. Psychol.* **2018**, *127*, 623–638. [CrossRef]
41. Deasy, C.; Coughlan, B.; Pironom, J.; Jourdan, D.; Mannix-McNamara, P. Psychological Distress and Coping Amongst Higher Education Students: A Mixed Method Enquiry. *PLoS ONE* **2014**, *9*, e115193. [CrossRef]
42. Hirshkowitz, M.; Whiton, K.; Albert, S.M.; Alessi, C.; Bruni, O.; DonCarlos, L.; Hazen, N.; Herman, J.; Adams Hillard, P.J.; Katz, E.S.; et al. National Sleep Foundation's Updated Sleep Duration Recommendations: Final Report. *Sleep Health* **2015**, *1*, 233–243. [CrossRef] [PubMed]
43. Carpi, M.; Cianfarani, C.; Vestri, A. Sleep Quality and Its Associations with Physical and Mental Health-Related Quality of Life among University Students: A Cross-Sectional Study. *Int. J. Environ. Res. Public Health* **2022**, *19*, 2874. [CrossRef]
44. Schmickler, J.M.; Blaschke, S.; Robbins, R.; Mess, F. Determinants of Sleep Quality: A Cross-Sectional Study in University Students. *Int. J. Environ. Res. Public Health* **2023**, *20*, 2019. [CrossRef] [PubMed]
45. Johansson, F.; Rozental, A.; Edlund, K.; Côté, P.; Sundberg, T.; Onell, C.; Rudman, A.; Skillgate, E. Associations between Procrastination and Subsequent Health Outcomes Among University Students in Sweden. *JAMA Netw. Open* **2023**, *6*, e2249346. [CrossRef]
46. Almojali, A.I.; Almalki, S.A.; Alothman, A.S.; Masuadi, E.M.; Alaqeel, M.K. The Prevalence and Association of Stress with Sleep Quality among Medical Students. *J. Epidemiol. Glob. Health* **2017**, *7*, 169–174. [CrossRef]
47. Kim, J.; Hwang, E.H.; Shin, S.; Kim, K.H. University Students' Sleep and Mental Health Correlates in South Korea. *Healthcare* **2022**, *10*, 1635. [CrossRef] [PubMed]
48. Almarzouki, A.F.; Mandili, R.L.; Salloom, J.; Kamal, L.K.; Alharthi, O.; Alharthi, S.; Khayyat, N.; Baglagel, A.M. The Impact of Sleep and Mental Health on Working Memory and Academic Performance: A Longitudinal Study. *Brain Sci.* **2022**, *12*, 1525. [CrossRef]
49. Winiger, E.A.; Hitchcock, L.N.; Bryan, A.D.; Cinnamon Bidwell, L. Cannabis Use and Sleep: Expectations, Outcomes, and the Role of Age. *Addict. Behav.* **2021**, *112*, 106642. [CrossRef]
50. Simons, J.S.; Correia, C.J.; Carey, K.B.; Borsari, B.E. Validating a Five Factor Marijuana Motives Measure: Relations with Use, Problems, and Alcohol Motives. *J. Couns. Psychol.* **1998**, *45*, 265–273. [CrossRef]
51. Sznitman, S.R.; Shochat, T.; van Rijswijk, L.; Greene, T.; Cousijn, J. Cannabis and Alcohol Use and Their Associations with Sleep: A Daily Diary Investigation of Single-Use and Co-Use in College Students. *Cannabis Cannabinoid Res.* **2023**, *8*, 527–536. [CrossRef]
52. Carballo-Fazanes, A.; Rico-Díaz, J.; Barcala-Furelos, R.; Rey, E.; Rodríguez-Fernández, J.E.; Varela-Casal, C.; Abelairas-Gómez, C. Physical Activity Habits and Determinants, Sedentary Behaviour and Lifestyle in University Students. *Int. J. Environ. Res. Public Health* **2020**, *17*, 3272. [CrossRef] [PubMed]
53. Knapstad, M.; Sivertsen, B.; Knudsen, A.K.; Smith, O.R.F.; Aarø, L.E.; Lønning, K.J.; Skogen, J.C. Trends in self-reported psychological distress among college and university students from 2010 to 2018. *Psychol. Med.* **2021**, *51*, 470–478. [CrossRef] [PubMed]
54. Li, W.; Yin, J.; Cai, X.; Cheng, X.; Wang, Y. Association between Sleep Duration and Quality and Depressive Symptoms Among University Students: A Cross-Sectional Study. *PLoS ONE* **2020**, *15*, e0238811. [CrossRef]
55. Steptoe, A.; Peacey, V.; Wardle, J. Sleep Duration and Health in Young Adults. *Arch. Intern. Med.* **2006**, *166*, 1689–1692. [CrossRef] [PubMed]

Disclaimer/Publisher's Note: The statements, opinions and data contained in all publications are solely those of the individual author(s) and contributor(s) and not of MDPI and/or the editor(s). MDPI and/or the editor(s) disclaim responsibility for any injury to people or property resulting from any ideas, methods, instructions or products referred to in the content.

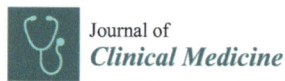

Article

Examining Anxiety and Insomnia in Internship Students and Their Association with Internet Gaming Disorder

Tahani K. Alshammari [1,*], Aleksandra M. Rogowska [2,*], Anan M. Alobaid [3], Noor W. Alharthi [3], Awatif B. Albaker [1] and Musaad A. Alshammari [1]

1. Department of Pharmacology and Toxicology, College of Pharmacy, King Saud University, Riyadh 11451, Saudi Arabia; abaker@ksu.edu.sa (A.B.A.); malshammari@ksu.edu.sa (M.A.A.)
2. Institute of Psychology, University of Opole, 45-052 Opole, Poland
3. College of Pharmacy, King Saud University, Riyadh 11451, Saudi Arabia; 438202720@student.ksu.edu.sa (A.M.A.); 438201681@student.ksu.edu.sa (N.W.A.)
* Correspondence: talshammary@ksu.edu.sa (T.K.A.); arogowska@uni.opole.pl (A.M.R.)

Abstract: Background: Internships are a mandatory graduation requirement to help medical students transition to the work environment. Some individuals are prone to anxiety in an unfamiliar environment, which is a public concern among young adults. Here, we investigated the mechanism between internet gaming disorder and anxiety and insomnia among internship students. **Methods:** A convenient sample of 267 internship students was collected in a cross-sectional study module between 17 July and 27 December 2022. The survey contained a 7-item Generalized Anxiety Disorder (GAD-7), Athens Insomnia Scale (AIS), and Internet Gaming Disorder Scale—Short-Form (IGDS9-SF). The association was estimated using Pearson's correlations, and network analysis was performed to characterize these associations. **Results:** Our results indicate that about 60% of participants exhibited mild to severe anxiety and insomnia, while 2.28% showed symptoms of internet gaming disorder. Also, we found a moderate association between anxiety and insomnia. An item-level analysis indicated that GAD_1 "feeling anxious" and GAD_5 "unable to sit still" are essential for gaming, and that GAD_2 "uncontrollable worrying" is crucial for insomnia. This indicated an interplay between these items, supported by our centrality analysis, where we found that GAD_1 and GAD_2 depicted high centrality. **Conclusions:** We found high rates of anxiety and insomnia in internship students and the association between selected symptoms of anxiety and insomnia. At the same time, low rates of internet gaming disorder could be attributed to a lack of time for entertainment and an increased awareness of its risks. Given these findings, an awareness of anxiety and insomnia risk should be emphasized.

Keywords: insomnia; anxiety; gaming disorder; intern students; mental health; network analysis

1. Introduction

Mental health disorders such as anxiety, depression, sleep difficulty, and addiction behavior are serious psychological and health problems. People living under stress, such as undergraduates and interns, are more subjected to such conditions [1]. Reports indicated a higher risk of developing anxiety and depression in undergraduate students in the first and second waves of the pandemic [2,3]. Further, the prevalence of depression during the second wave of COVID-19 was documented as high as 50% in cross-sectional settings [4], indicating the rate of psychological stress has been elevated since the pandemic. In line with this, a two-year longitudinal post-COVID-19 pandemic study examined the trajectories of mental health aspects in the Italian population. The study indicated a reduction in depression, anxiety, and sleep disturbances. However, the duration of evening sleep was gradually reduced in young individuals [5].

The internship is a transition phase where students acquire practical experience and become familiar with the work environment [6]. Internships during the final undergraduate year strongly dictate the professional transition to practice and employment [7]. Interns had a higher prevalence of psychological distress when compared to the general population [8]. Psychological conditions could cause changes in behaviors and personality. These changes could be driven by the long working hours associated with continuous sleep deprivation [9]. Other challenges interns face are adjustment issues and building their professional competence, which includes interpersonal and communication skills, knowledge, experience, adapting to a decision-making role, difficulty with the licensure exam, and job pursuit [8,10].

Online gaming has become a public health concern among young adults, as it can lead to addiction. Excessive online gaming is becoming a behavior pattern that causes harmful consequences at physiological and psychological levels. This behavior can be severe enough to damage personal, family, social, educational, occupational, and other critical aspects of functioning [11]. As various studies show a high prevalence of anxiety and insomnia among intern students [12–14], it is essential to understand the particular pattern of anxiety and insomnia associations in relation to online gaming.

Insomnia is a common sleep disorder characterized by difficulty falling or staying asleep, usually accompanied by daytime impairment [4]. Chronic sleep restriction is linked to daytime cognitive deficit, metabolic dysfunction, and alterations in the endocrine system [15]. Further, insomnia is related to somatization and emotional dysregulation [16]. Also, a volumetric analysis of the brains of patients with anxiety disorder showed abnormalities in magnetic resonance readout, and these alterations were associated with the severity of insomnia [17].

It has been reported that insomnia is higher among older people, females, and people with medical and psychiatric conditions [4]. However, research studies and reviews have highlighted the prevalence of insomnia and sleep deprivation in residents and interns [12,18–20]. In line with this, a survey-based report showed that short sleep duration was associated with anxiety during the internship, and predicted future anxiety symptoms [12].

We previously reported, using regression and mediation models, that anxiety and insomnia mediate gaming addiction and depression association [21]. In another report, we found that health sciences college students exhibited a higher level of anxiety; more than 50% of the participants reported moderate to severe anxiety [22]. Further, in the second wave of COVID-19, we found a significant number of college students were at risk of anxiety and depression, and there was an association between these risks and poor sleep quality [23]. We further examined the risks of insomnia in Saudi students, and more than 70% of the participants were at higher risk of experiencing insomnia while addressing the Athens Insomnia Scale [24].

A two-year longitudinal study indicated more than a third of college students exhibited insomnia, and those with psychological determinants, including perfectionism and low self-esteem, were predisposed to it [25]. In line with this, another report examining the mental well-being of undergraduate nursing students indicated that more than 70% of the participants exhibited higher risks of insomnia [26]. Also, a study conducted at Bielefeld University reported that more than 70% of the study participants presented insomnia symptoms [27]. Further, students with insomnia reported clinical and non-clinical conditions, including anxiety, depression, stress, and fatigue [28–30]. Thus, the relationship between insomnia and mental health issues is well acknowledged. Further, insomnia is associated with addiction [31,32] and alcohol use [33,34], indicating an intervention is paramount at the organizational level to raise awareness about the clinical consequences of insomnia.

Reports have indicated that the severity of internet gaming disorder is linked to anxiety and poor sleep quality [35–37]. Fazeli et al. [38] found a mechanistic indication that anxiety is a significant mediator of insomnia and internet gaming disorder. Yet, these reports were based on total scores, which makes it difficult to intervene and target a specific symptom.

Network analysis is an emerging tool for understanding the complex relations of mental disorders' comorbidities. The structural foundation is a dimensional module composed of nodes and edges. Nodes represent symptoms, while edges reflect the relationship between these nodes. This analysis module would determine the most influential–central–symptom, identifying an appropriate symptom-based intervention [39,40].

In the context of psychiatric disorders, network analysis has been utilized to delineate the comorbid symptoms of anxiety and depression [41–44], depression and psychological factors [45,46], eating disorders, and psychiatric diseases [47]. Yet, most of these reports were conducted during the COVID-19 pandemic. Additionally, only a few studies examined insomnia and anxiety. However, these studies included other conditions and factors, such as depression and workload [48–50]. The existence of additional multivariates could add further heterogeneity to the insomnia–anxiety network analysis [39].

In a clinical setting, anxiety and insomnia are linked to economic, social, and cultural components [51–55]. Thus, findings from studies conducted in Africa, North and South Asia, and Western countries might not be applicable. Even though interns face challenges of novel and stressful training environments along with maintaining sufficient sleep hours, a comprehensive study examining this sample population has not been conducted. As far as we know, no studies based on network analysis at an item-level analysis examined the anxiety–insomnia–gaming network in the internship sample population. Also, none have been established in Middle Eastern countries. Here, we aimed to explore the complex relationships between the symptoms of insomnia, anxiety, and internet gaming disorder among internship students using network analysis.

2. Materials and Methods

A cross-sectional study was conducted on male and female internship-year students from King Saud University from 17 July to 27 December 2022. An online survey was generated by Google Forms in Arabic and English and distributed to participants using convenient sampling technology through Twitter, WhatsApp, and Telegram. An electronic consent notification, indicating that the participant agrees to participate in the study and that the response is entirely confidential and voluntary, along with a clear indication of the objectives and descriptions of the project, was shown at the beginning of the survey. Ethical approval was obtained from the Institutional Review Board at King Saud University (KSU), Riyadh, Saudi Arabia (Ref No. 22/0055/IRB), approved on the 23rd of January 2022. Although 267 students responded to invitations, four were excluded because of missing data, totaling more than 5%. Finally, the data of 263 participants were statistically analyzed.

2.1. Participants

A total of 263 students, aged between 18 and 30 ($M = 22.83$, $SD = 1.37$), participated in the study, including 67.68% ($n = 178$) of females and 32.32% ($n = 85$) of males, 95.82% ($n = 252$) of singles and 4.18% ($n = 11$) of married (Table 1). The number of family members at home ranged between 1 and 14, with a mean of 6 ($M = 6.41$, $SD = 2.35$). The participants in the study were interns who were studying at Saudi institutes from different colleges, which include the college of pharmacy ($n = 55$, 20.91%), college of dentistry ($n = 18$, 6.84%), college of medicine ($n = 10$, 3.80%), college of nursing ($n = 41$, 15.59%), college of applied medical sciences ($n = 120$, 45.63%), and college of humanities ($n = 2$, 0.76%).

2.2. Measurements

2.2.1. Anxiety

The Generalized Anxiety Disorder (GAD-7) scale is a validated 7-item used widely and easily to screen for anxiety in general and research settings [56]. The GAD-7 scale uses a four-point Likert scale from 0 (not at all) to 3 (every day), with total scores ranging from 0 to 21; higher scores represent higher grades of anxiety. The total scores of 5, 10, and 15 are taken as the cut-off points for mild, moderate, and severe anxiety, respectively. Both

English, Cronbach's alpha = 0.92 [57], and Arabic, Cronbach's alpha = 0.95 [58] versions of this tool were used in the study.

Table 1. Demographic characteristics of students (N = 263).

Variable	Category	n/M	%/SD
Age	Range 18–30	22.83	1.37
Sex	Male	85	32.319
	Female	178	67.681
Relationship status	Single	252	95.817
	Married	11	4.183
Number of family members	Range 1–14	6.41	2.35
Internship program—college -	Applied medical sciences	120	45.63
	Medicine	10	3.8
	Dentistry	18	6.84
	Nursing	41	15.59
	Pharmacy	55	20.91
	Humanities	2	0.76

2.2.2. Insomnia

The Athens Insomnia Scale (AIS) is an 8-item questionnaire developed to assess insomnia, demonstrating strong consistency, reliability, and validity [59]. The first five items assess problems with sleep induction, awakening during the night, early morning awakening, total sleep duration, and overall sleep quality. The last three items are about the next-day consequences of insomnia, such as problems with a sense of well-being, functioning, and sleepiness during the day. Each AIS item is scored on a 0-to-3 scale, with 0 representing no problem and 3 representing a profoundly serious problem. The overall score on these eight items varied from 0 to 24, with a score of AIS $\geq$ 6 indicating insomnia. Subjects were asked to rate positively if they had experienced the item at least thrice weekly in the previous month. Both English, Cronbach's alpha = 0.84 [60], and Arabic, Cronbach's alpha = 0.83 [61] versions of this tool were used in the study.

2.2.3. Gaming

The Internet Gaming Disorder Scale 9—Short-Form (IGDS9-SF) is the most commonly used psychometric tool for evaluating the severity of an internet gaming disorder over a year [62,63]. The IGDS9-SF incorporates all nine internet gaming disorder criteria established by the American Psychiatric Association (APA) in the DSM-5, with attributes of conciseness and short administration time, making it useful in clinical and research settings. Furthermore, the IGDS9-SF's psychometric properties, including internal consistency and validity, have been thoroughly evaluated [64]. The scale uses a 5-point Likert-type: Never (1), Rarely (2), Sometimes (3), Often (4), and Very Often (5). The total score is calculated by summing the nine items (range: 9–45), with a higher score indicating a higher level of internet gaming disorder (IGD). A response of "Very often" on five or more of the nine items on the IGDS9-SF is considered indicative of IGD [65]. Both English, Cronbach's alpha = 0.91 [65], and Arabic, Cronbach's alpha = 0.92 [66] versions of this tool were used in the study.

2.3. Demographics

The demographic characteristics assessed in the study are participants' age, gender, marital status, number of family members at home, and internship program.

2.4. Statistical Analysis

Descriptive statistics were performed to examine the parametric properties of variables, including range of scores, mean (M), standard deviation (SD), skewness, and kurtosis.

Reliability was assessed using Cronbach's α coefficients. Pearson's correlation analysis was conducted to examine associations between internet gaming disorder, anxiety, and insomnia symptoms. Finally, the network analysis (NA) was implemented to identify the most important variables for the model of associations between particular symptoms of insomnia, general anxiety disorder, and internet gaming disorder among internship students. We used the NA with extended Bayesian information criteria and graphical least absolute shrinkage, and selection operator (EBICglasso) as an estimator. The weighted network between nodes is represented by magnitude (the thicker the lines between nodes, the stronger the relationship). The closeness between nodes also shows the strength of correlations. Closeness centrality quantifies how close a node is to all other nodes in the network. It is calculated as the inverse of the sum of the shortest path distances between a node and all other nodes in the network. Several centrality indices (i.e., betweenness, closeness, degree, and expected influence) identified the network model's most relevant, influential, and crucial variables. All statistical tests were performed using the JASP ver. 0.16.1.0. software for Windows.

3. Results

3.1. Prevalence of Internet Gaming Disorder, Anxiety, and Insomnia Symptoms

About 87 of our participants responded to the Arabic questionnaire, and 167 responded to the English version. The frequencies of particular categories of disordered symptoms are shown in Table 1. Among participants, only six (2.28%) students met the criteria of gaming addiction (i.e., a minimum of 5 out of 9 items of the IGDS9-SF rated as "very often"). Moderate or severe symptoms of general anxiety disorder (GAD-7 $\geq$ 10) were found in 28.90% of participants (see Table 2 for more details). Most of the interns (60%) presented insomnia symptoms (AIS $\geq$ 6).

Table 2. Frequencies of particular categories of internet gaming disorder, anxiety, and insomnia symptoms.

Variable	Categories	n	%
Internet gaming disorder	Non-disordered gamers	257	97.72
	Disordered gamers	6	2.28
Generalized anxiety disorder	No symptoms	92	34.98
	Mild symptoms	95	36.12
	Moderate symptoms	54	20.53
	Severe symptoms	22	8.37
Insomnia	No insomnia	104	39.54
	Insomnia	159	60.46

Note. Disordered gamers can be identified if they respond "Very often" to at least five of the nine items on the IGDS9-SF. Insomnia is considered with a score of six or more in the AIS.

3.2. Associations between Internet Gaming Disorder, Anxiety, and Insomnia Symptoms

Descriptive statistics are presented in Table 3. Since the sample size was quite large (N > 200), and skewness and kurtosis ranged between +0.50, the properties of internet gaming disorder, general anxiety disorder, and insomnia symptoms were appropriate for further parametric statistical tests.

Table 3. Descriptive statistics (N = 263).

Variable	Range	M	SD	Skewness	Kurtosis	Cronbach's α
Internet gaming disorder	9–41	18.53	7.84	0.64	−0.49	0.89
Anxiety	0–21	7.22	5.06	0.56	−0.32	0.89
Insomnia	0–23	7.06	4.52	0.52	−0.03	0.83

A Pearson's correlation analysis showed that internet gaming disorder is related to anxiety symptoms, $r = 0.35$, [95% CI (0.24, 0.45)], $p < 0.001$ (small strength). Insomnia symptoms are linked to internet gaming disorder, $r = 0.27$, [95% CI (0.16, 0.38)], $p < 0.001$ (small strength). Also, a moderate association was found between general anxiety disorder and insomnia symptoms, $r = 0.61$, [95% CI (0.50, 0.70)], $p < 0.001$. All associations were positive (see Figure 1).

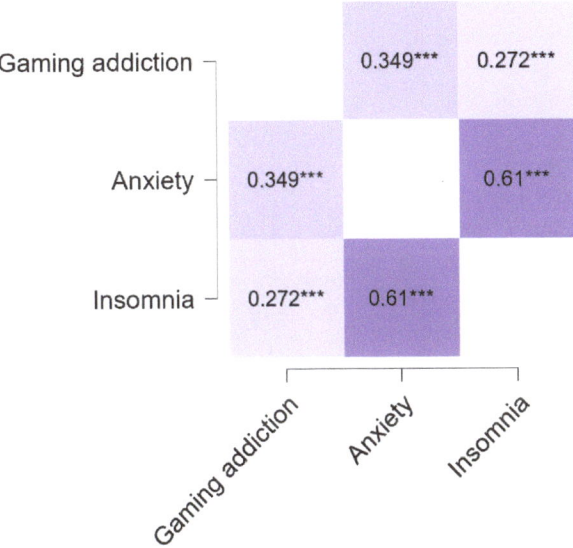

Figure 1. Pearson's correlations between internet gaming disorder, anxiety, and insomnia symptoms ($N = 263$). *** $p < 0.001$.

3.3. Network Analysis

The network analysis was performed to examine the complex relationships between particular symptoms of insomnia, anxiety, and internet gaming disorder among internship students. The structure of associations is presented in Figure 2. Our findings indicated a positive relationship association, and they indicated that a peripheral cluster existed within the internet gaming disorder scale. It is composed of IGDS_1, "the preoccupation with online/offline gaming" IGDS_3, "the need to spend increasing amounts of time engaged in games" IGDS_4, "unsuccessful attempts to control participation in games", and the IGDS_2, "experience of unpleasant symptoms when gaming is taken away" nodes.

Another connection was detected between IGDS_5, "loss of interest in previous hobbies", IGDS_6, "continued excessive use of games despite knowledge of psychosocial problems", and IGDS_9, "jeopardizing or losing a significant relationship, job, or education opportunity because of participation in games", nodes. A moderate association was observed between IGDS_3, "the need to spend increasing amounts of time engaged in the games" node, and IGDS_8, "the node of use of games to escape or relieve negative moods".

The nodes GAD_1, "feeling nervous", and GAD_2, "uncontrollable worrying", were strongly connected. The nodes GAD_3, "worrying too much", and GAD_4, " trouble relaxing", were strongly clustered. A direct association was observed between GAD_5 "restlessness" and GAD_6 "irritability" nodes.

The insomnia network indicated a strong association between AIS_2 "awakening problems" and AIS_3 "awakening earlier than desired" nodes. Similarly, the nodes of AIS_4, "sense of sleep duration sufficiency", and AIS_5, "satisfaction of sleep quality", were interconnected. Additionally, the nodes of AIS_6, "sense of well-being during the day", and AIS_7, "physical and mental functioning during the day", were strongly connected.

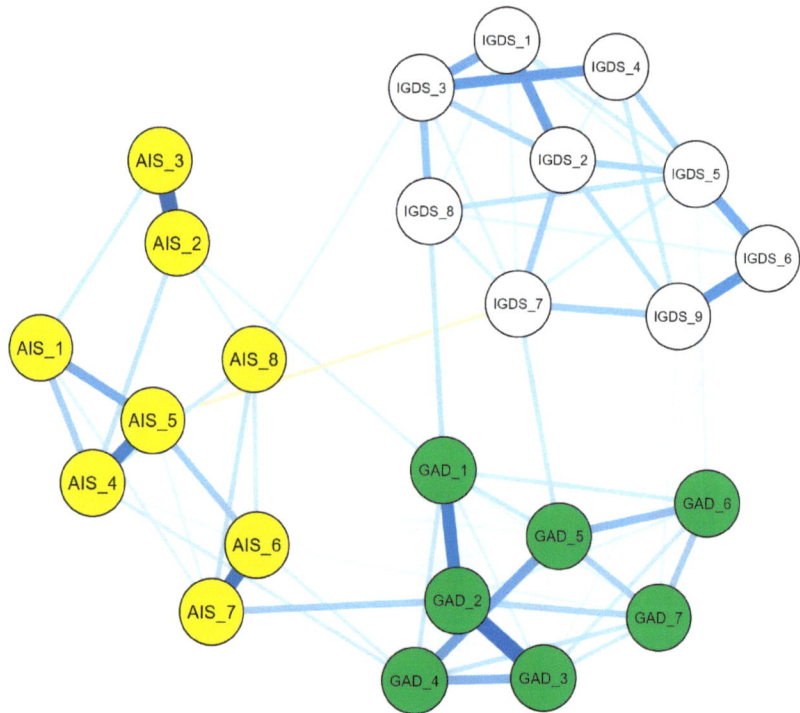

Figure 2. Network structure of associations between the insomnia (AIS), anxiety (GAD), and gaming disorder (IGDS) scales. Note. The blue line represents a positive relationship, while the orange line indicates a negative association between nodes in the network model. AIS = Athens Insomnia Scale, AIS_1 = delaying sleep, AIS_2 = problems with waking during the night, AIS_3 = final awakening earlier than desired, AIS_4 = sense of total sleep duration sufficiency, AIS_5 = overall satisfaction of sleep quality, AIS_6 = sense of well-being during the day, AIS_7 = physical and mental functioning during the day, AIS_8 = sleepiness during the day. GAD = General Anxiety Disorder, GAD_1 = feeling nervous, anxious, or on edge, GAD_2 = not being able to stop or control worrying, GAD_3 = worrying too much about different things, GAD_4 = trouble relaxing, GAD_5 = being so restless that it is hard to sit still, GAD_6 = becoming easily annoyed or irritable, GAD_7 = feeling afraid as if something awful might happen. IGDS = Internet Gaming Disorder Scale, IGDS_1 = preoccupation with online/offline gaming, IGDS_2 = experience of unpleasant symptoms when gaming is taken away, IGDS_3 = the need to spend increasing amounts of time engaged in games, IGDS_4 = unsuccessful attempts to control participation in games, IGDS_5 = loss of interest in previous hobbies and entertainment as a result of, and with the exception of, games, IGDS_6 = continued excessive use of games despite knowledge of psychosocial problems, IGDS_7 = deceiving family members, therapists, or others regarding the amount of gaming, IGDS_8 = use of games to escape or relieve negative moods, IGDS_9 = jeopardizing or losing a significant relationship, job, or education or career opportunity because of participation in games.

With the IGDS-GAD model, IGDS_8, "the use of games to escape or relieve negative moods", and GAD_1, "the feeling nervous" nodes, had the strongest connection. Another direct positive connection was detected between GAD_5, "the restlessness" node, and IGDS_7, "the deceiving family members or others regarding the amount of gaming" node.

With the AIS-GAD model, the nodes of AIS_6 "sense of well-being during the day", and AIS_4 "sense of sleep duration sufficiency" were directly connected to GAD_4 "trouble relaxing". Also, the node of AIS_7 "physical and mental functioning during the day" was directly connected to the GAD_2 node. Another direct positive connection was detected between the GAD_1 "feeling nervous" and AIS_2 "awakening problems" nodes.

With the AIS-IGDS model, a negative association was detected between the AIS_5 "satisfaction of sleep quality" node and IGDS_7 "deceiving family members or others regarding the amount of gaming" node.

Figure 3 depicts the centrality plot, and Supplementary Table S1 exhibits the centrality analysis values. Our analysis indicated that IGDS_7, "deceiving family members or others regarding the amount of gaming", is more critical for betweenness centrality. Nodes with high closeness centrality can quickly interact with other nodes in the network. In the present study, IGDS_7 and GAD_1 are critical for closeness centrality. In addition, GAD_2 determines the degree and expected influence of centrality.

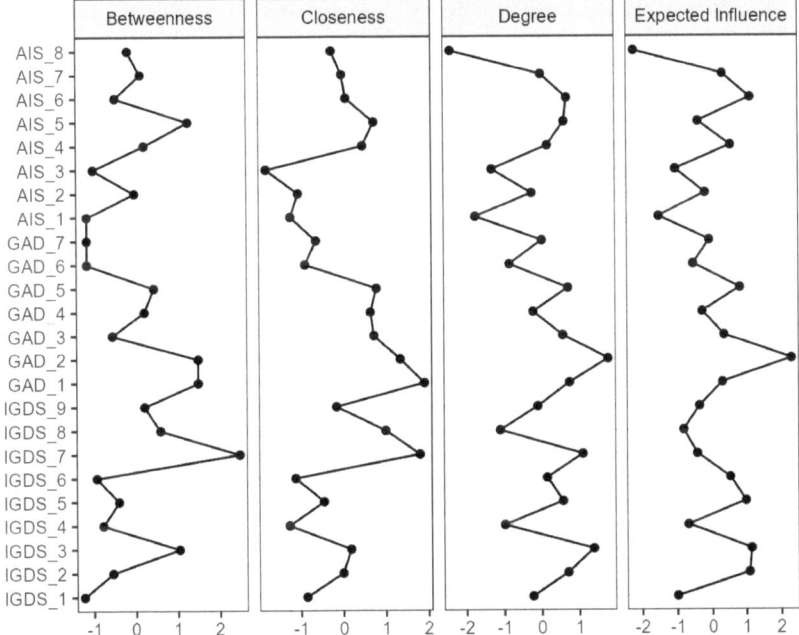

Figure 3. Centrality plot. Note. AIS = Athens Insomnia Scale, AIS_1 = delaying sleep, AIS_2 = problems with waking during the night, AIS_3 = final awakening earlier than desired, AIS_4 = sense of total sleep duration sufficiency, AIS_5 = overall satisfaction of sleep quality, AIS_6 = sense of well-being during the day, AIS_7 = physical and mental functioning during the day, AIS_8 = sleepiness during the day. GAD = General Anxiety Disorder, GAD_1 = feeling nervous, anxious, or on edge, GAD_2 = not being able to stop or control worrying, GAD_3 = worrying too much about different things, GAD_4 = trouble relaxing, GAD_5 = being so restless that it is hard to sit still, GAD_6 = becoming easily annoyed or irritable, GAD_7 = feeling afraid as if something awful might happen. IGDS = Internet Gaming Disorder Scale, IGDS_1 = preoccupation with online/offline gaming, IGDS_2 = experience of unpleasant symptoms when gaming is taken away, IGDS_3 = the need to spend increasing amounts of time engaged in games, IGDS_4 = unsuccessful attempts to control participation in games, IGDS_5 = loss of interest in previous hobbies and entertainment as a result of, and with the exception of, games, IGDS_6 = continued excessive use of games despite knowledge of psychosocial problems, IGDS_7 = deceiving family members, therapists, or others regarding the amount of gaming, IGDS_8 = use of games to escape or relieve negative moods, IGDS_9 = jeopardizing or losing a significant relationship, job, or education or career opportunity because of participation in games.

4. Discussion

Network analysis is a novel approach to understand the complex interactions between symptoms and conditions. In the context of the anxiety–insomnia–gaming network, the analysis can identify which symptoms are most strongly interconnected and how they may be contributing to each other's severity. In this work, we found elevated rates of anxiety and insomnia in internship students. A small percentage of our study participants exhibited gaming addiction. Further, we identified an association between selected symptoms of the anxiety–insomnia–gaming network. The item-level analysis indicated that GAD_1, "feeling anxious", and GAD_5, "restlessness", are central to gaming and that GAD_2, "uncontrollable worrying", is central to insomnia. This indicates an interplay between these items, supported by our centrality analysis, where we found that GAD_1 and GAD_2 depicted high centrality.

The rates of anxiety and insomnia are high compared to the reported findings of existing studies. For instance, the prevalence of anxiety in the adult population is about 19% [67], whereas epidemiological-based studies indicated that the prevalence of insomnia is 21–25% [68]. Further, Perlis et al. [69] reported that around 30% of the population develop acute incidents of insomnia. Our findings indicated that about 2% showed symptoms of internet gaming disorder; a meta-analysis study reported that gaming disorder's global prevalence is around 3% [70], suggesting that the gaming pattern of our study sample aligns with its global prevalence.

Our Pearson's correlation findings indicated a significant association between insomnia and anxiety. In support of this, the association has been verified using multiple approaches [71–73]. A previous longitudinal report conducted in Switzerland indicated that repeated brief insomnia and continued insomnia were significantly linked to anxiety in young individuals (21–23 years). Further, the risk of insomnia reoccurrence was reasonably high [74]. Additionally, this association could lead to significant clinical consequences. For instance, functional Magnetic Resonance Imaging (fMRI) in anxiety–insomnia patients compared to healthy controls revealed a hyperactive posterior cingulate cortex and elevated network segregation. This elevation was significantly linked to the severity of insomnia [75]. In line with this, elevated functional connectivity was detected in the limbic system (amygdala) of patients diagnosed with primary insomnia [76]. Meanwhile, the amygdala is physiologically linked to emotional regulation [77].

A higher rate of insomnia could be attributed to multiple factors. College students, in particular, are at higher risk of acquiring insomnia, primarily due to social, academic, and professional concerns [78]. Mbous et al. reported that insomnia coexists in more than 70% of depressed students [79], indicating that having mood disorders elevates the risk of experiencing insomnia. An epidemiological study conducted on Portuguese adolescents concluded that female gender and age are substantial risk factors for acquiring insomnia [80], and a significant number of our study participants are female. In line with this, a study reported that experiencing one month of insomnia over one year was correlated inversely with age; the probability was higher in participants in their twenties and reduced compared to individuals in their thirties, then declined compared to participants in their forties. The study also indicated that insomnia is more prevalent in women [81].

A study conducted in multiple primary healthcare centers in Saudi populations from the Jeddah district concluded that severe insomnia is prevalent in younger individuals [82]. Additionally, a recent report indicated that adolescent females exhibited a higher prevalence of insomnia compared to males and younger-aged females. The report also showed that a higher prevalence of sleep reduction was linked to sleep hygiene practices, including caffeine consumption [83]. Another report on Saudi female college students indicated that coffee consumption exceeded 80% [84]. In support of this, another study on Saudi adolescents reported that 94% consumed coffee and caffeinated products [85], which could be a critical factor in the elevated rates of insomnia in Saudi college students.

Further, the Saudi lifestyle may contribute to these findings. With its dry and hot weather, Saudi Arabia may seem dormant. But as the sun sets, a remarkable transformation occurs. The cities burst into life, offering a vibrant and energetic nightlife starkly contrasting with the daytime heat. The cities are full of glowing shopping centers. Further, Arabian culture values coffee, and coffee shops are everywhere and always crowded with people. Additionally, the majority of family gatherings, weddings, and social events are carried out during the night [86].

The elevated level of insomnia could be clinically relevant to the risks of developing depression [87], heart disease [88], obesity [89], and cognitive dysfunction [90]. For instance, symptoms of insomnia have been identified as a predictive risk of depression and high blood pressure. In an eight-year follow-up cohort study, it was found that individuals exhibiting four symptoms of insomnia develop both depression and elevated blood pressure [91]. In line with this, studies from the early seventies documented changes in the rapid eye movement sleep latencies in depressed patients [87,92]. Further, a report indicated that the prevalence of type 2 diabetes is more than 20% in individuals with insomnia [93]. These clinical implications of insomnia highlight the need to establish an early intervention and/or preventive measures for insomnia.

The most predominant findings within our anxiety–insomnia–gaming network structure indicated that: (1) GAD_1 and GAD_2 are interconnected at a high centrality level; (2) GAD_2 is crucial for insomnia; (3) the GAD_3 cluster was most substantial among anxiety symptoms; (4) GAD_1 and GAD_5 are essential for internet gaming disorder; (5) the centrality analysis highlighted multiple nodes; those that project the most are IGDS_7, GAD_1, and GAD_2.

The item-level analysis found that GAD_1 and GAD_2 are interconnected at a high centrality level. Extended thinking and worrying have been linked to psychiatric [42,44] and behavioral conditions [94]. For example, a previous report indicated that GAD_1 intertwined with multiple domains of depression [44]. This connection could be established, as feeling nervous and being unable to control worrying are mirrors of persistent nervousness, which is a core symptom of anxiety [95].

Our findings highlighted GAD_3 as a central domain of the analysis, which could be partially driven by career entry worries [96]. Being worried too much is an essential symptom of anxiety disorder [95]. Previous research indicated that worrying too much is the central node of the depression–anxiety network in adolescents. Further, the study identified GAD_3 as a potential interventional target in adolescent individuals to mitigate the risk of the clinical consequences of depressive and anxiety symptoms [43], signifying the role of GAD_3 as a core symptom of anxiety.

Further, we found that GAD_2 "uncontrollable worrying" is crucial for insomnia. In a study examining anxiety–depression–insomnia, uncontrollable worrying was found to be a predominant node [97], which supports prior findings on the significant association between anxiety and insomnia [45,49,98]. Notably, a cross-sectional study has found that the severity index of insomnia is a predictive factor in developing psychiatric symptoms through extensive worrying and rumination [16].

Moreover, GAD_1, "feeling anxious", and GAD_5, "restlessness", are essential for internet gaming disorder. We found a direct link between IGDS_7 "deceiving family members regarding the amount of gaming" and GAD_1, and a connection between the IGDS_8, "use of games to escape or relieve negative moods", and GAD_5 nodes. Both GAD_1 and GAD_5 are essential for internet gaming disorder and are supported by the literature as key symptoms of anxiety that are essential for other mental conditions [42]. Additionally, GAD_5 is a core psychomotor symptom of anxiety [95]. A systematic review demonstrated that behavioral addiction, including gaming and gambling, was driven by poor emotional regulation. These behavioral addictions were mediated by seeking an escape from negative emotions [99]. Further, in adolescents, emotional regulation is directly linked to the time spent on gaming [100], even though, in our sample, the risk of exhibiting internet gaming disorder is minimal. This finding could be crucial for understanding the factors correlated with gaming addiction and considering that video gamers promote elevated levels of stress, loneliness, anxiety, depression, and alcohol use disorder [101].

Most of the existing literature utilizes network analysis on the general population using survey-based studies, which highlights the risk of developing a psychiatric disorder [42,43,46,48]. It has also been used for randomized controlled trial studies. For example, a previous report examined the impact of cognitive behavioral therapy on symptoms of insomnia and depression using network analysis. The study findings indicated a sequential improvement in insomnia symptoms driven by cognitive behavioral therapy in depressed individuals. These improvements started in the first week of treatment, with early morning awakening symptoms depicted by the Insomnia Severity Index scale, and the improvement in individuals' dissatisfaction symptoms was reached by the fourth week of treatment [102]. Another translational aspect of employing network analysis in psychopathology is examining behavioral and biological connectivity. This clinical analysis has been utilized in a study investigating the connectivity of peripartum depression and the biological markers of stress and reproduction. Item-level analysis indicated that dislike—estriol, fear—a corticotropin-releasing hormone, cry—cortisol, and loneliness—cortisol were interconnected in depressed pregnant Latina women [103]. Therefore, it is for future studies to translate these findings by establishing a biochemical association, such as the cortisol serum level, or by interview-based psychological assessment.

It is worth mentioning that previous studies examined the association between insomnia and anxiety. However, this is the first report to examine insomnia and anxiety in an item-based analysis with respect to gaming addiction. This is also the first report to examine this association in an internship sample population. One interesting finding was the lesser prevalence of gaming addiction in our sample. Most importantly, our findings indicated that "feeling anxious", "restlessness", and "uncontrollable worrying" are central symptoms in this association. Therefore, a key implication is needed for studies translating this knowledge via behavioral strategies to target these disturbances [104–106]. Another intervention method is establishing a campus-based counseling program. A support group consisting of experts and peer students would facilitate the student's stress coping and understanding of their feelings [107–109].

Our findings of the anxiety–insomnia–gaming network align with contemporary studies that have identified Dysregulation of Mood, Energy, and Social Rhythms Syndrome (DYMERS) [110,111]. The DYMER syndrome is clinically significant in the progression of health conditions. For example, exposure to stress represents a risk factor for the bipolar spectrum [112]. Further, DYMER is manifested by the dysregulation of behavioral, social, and biological rhythms such as sleep, stress, diet, eating habits, and sociability [110,111,113]. These studies highlighted the research gaps in social and behavioral rhythmic domain dysregulation.

Limitations of the study: While the study at hand is novel and significant, with network analysis providing a comprehensive profiling of the study elements, it is crucial to acknowledge the presence of certain limitations. The study design, for instance, is cross-sectional. Although commonly used, this design limits the ability to establish a causal interface between the study variables. Secondly, the sample was collected via convenient snowball sampling. Random sampling could overcome sample and study bias representation. Additionally, it is important to note that recall bias is a potential factor that cannot be entirely ruled out. The influence of self and social desirability on participant responses could impact the validity of the study's findings.

Furthermore, anxiety and insomnia are highly comorbid and affected by physiological and psychological health conditions, and we did not include any clinical variables within the study. Finally, network analysis is promising, and emerging in the context of psychiatric and psychological studies. Yet, studies examining the accuracy and stability of this analysis framework are sparse [114]. Future studies should consider these limitations using a prospective longitudinal cohort within a larger sample size.

5. Conclusions

We found high rates of anxiety and insomnia, and an association between selected symptoms of anxiety and insomnia. The Saudi lifestyle may contribute to these findings. Low gaming addiction rates could be attributed to a lack of entertainment time and increased risk awareness. Deliberation anxiety–insomnia–gaming network domains are beneficial in identifying proper psychological and functional interventions. Given these findings, an awareness of anxiety and insomnia risks should be emphasized.

Supplementary Materials: The following supporting information can be downloaded at: https://www.mdpi.com/article/10.3390/jcm13144054/s1, Table S1: Centrality measures per variable.

Author Contributions: Conceptualization, T.K.A., A.M.R. and M.A.A.; methodology, T.K.A. and A.M.R.; formal analysis, A.M.R.; investigation, A.M.A., N.W.A. and A.B.A.; resources, T.K.A.; writing—original draft preparation A.B.A., A.M.A., N.W.A., T.K.A. and A.M.R.; writing—review and editing, T.K.A., M.A.A. and A.M.R.; supervision, T.K.A. and A.B.A.; project administration, M.A.A. All authors have read and agreed to the published version of the manuscript.

Funding: This research received no external funding.

Institutional Review Board Statement: Ethical approval was granted by the Institutional Review Board at King Saud University in Riyadh, Saudi Arabia (Ref No. 22/0055/IRB).

Informed Consent Statement: At the beginning of the survey, participants were provided with a consent participation message, a description of the project aims, and reassurance that their responses were confidential and completely voluntary.

Data Availability Statement: Data are available upon reasonable request.

Acknowledgments: The authors extend their appreciation to the College of Pharmacy Research Center, Deanship of Scientific Research, King Saud University.

Conflicts of Interest: The authors declare no conflicts of interest.

References

1. Wu, T.; Jia, X.; Shi, H.; Niu, J.; Yin, X.; Xie, J.; Wang, X. Prevalence of mental health problems during the COVID-19 pandemic: A systematic review and meta-analysis. *J. Affect. Disord.* **2021**, *281*, 91–98. [CrossRef] [PubMed]
2. Odriozola-González, P.; Planchuelo-Gómez, Á.; Irurtia, M.J.; de Luis-García, R. Psychological effects of the COVID-19 outbreak and lockdown among students and workers of a Spanish university. *Psychiatry Res.* **2020**, *290*, 113108. [CrossRef] [PubMed]
3. Rogowska, A.M.; Kuśnierz, C.; Pavlova, I.; Chilicka, K. A Path Model for Subjective Well-Being during the Second Wave of the COVID-19 Pandemic: A Comparative Study among Polish and Ukrainian University Students. *J. Clin. Med.* **2022**, *11*, 4726. [CrossRef] [PubMed]
4. Oh, C.M.; Kim, H.Y.; Na, H.K.; Cho, K.H.; Chu, M.K. The Effect of Anxiety and Depression on Sleep Quality of Individuals with High Risk for Insomnia: A Population-Based Study. *Front. Neurol.* **2019**, *10*, 849. [CrossRef] [PubMed]
5. Salfi, F.; Amicucci, G.; Corigliano, D.; Viselli, L.; D'Atri, A.; Tempesta, D.; Gorgoni, M.; Scarpelli, S.; Alfonsi, V.; Ferrara, M. Two years after lockdown: Longitudinal trajectories of sleep disturbances and mental health over the COVID-19 pandemic, and the effects of age, gender and chronotype. *J. Sleep Res.* **2023**, *32*, e13767. [CrossRef] [PubMed]
6. Weible, R. Are Universities Reaping the Available Benefits Internship Programs Offer? *J. Educ. Bus.* **2009**, *85*, 59–63. [CrossRef]
7. Matthew, S.M.; Taylor, R.M.; Ellis, R.A. Relationships between students' experiences of learning in an undergraduate internship programme and new graduates' experiences of professional practice. *High. Educ.* **2012**, *64*, 529–542. [CrossRef]
8. Naidu, K.; Torline, J.R.; Henry, M.; Thornton, H.B. Depressive symptoms and associated factors in medical interns at a tertiary hospital. *S. Afr. J. Psychiatr.* **2019**, *25*, 1322. [CrossRef] [PubMed]
9. Rosen, I.M.; Gimotty, P.A.; Shea, J.A.; Bellini, L.M. Evolution of Sleep Quantity, Sleep Deprivation, Mood Disturbances, Empathy, and Burnout among Interns. *Acad. Med.* **2006**, *81*, 82–85. [CrossRef]
10. Yi, Q.-F.; Yan, J.; Zhang, C.-J.; Yang, G.-L.; Huang, H.; Yang, Y. The experience of anxiety among Chinese undergraduate nursing students in the later period of their internships: Findings from a qualitative study. *BMC Nurs.* **2022**, *21*, 70. [CrossRef]
11. Yarasani, P.; Shaik, R.; Myla, A. Prevalence of addiction to online video games: Gaming disorder among medical students. *Int. J. Community Med. Public Health* **2018**, *5*, 4237. [CrossRef]
12. Kalmbach, D.A.; Abelson, J.L.; Arnedt, J.T.; Zhao, Z.; Schubert, J.R.; Sen, S. Insomnia symptoms and short sleep predict anxiety and worry in response to stress exposure: A prospective cohort study of medical interns. *Sleep Med.* **2019**, *55*, 40–47. [CrossRef]
13. Merchant, H.; Nayak, A.; Mulkalwar, A. A study to assess the prevalence of depression, anxiety and stress among interns across the State of Maharashtra, India. *Indian J. Ment. Health* **2018**, *5*, 184–190. [CrossRef]

14. Nooli, A.; Asiri, A.; Asiri, A.; Alqarni, M.; Alhilali, F.; Alayafi, M. Prevalence of depression among medical interns in King Khalid University. *Int. J. Med. Res. Prof.* **2017**, *3*, 131–133.
15. Banks, S.; Dinges, D.F. Behavioral and physiological consequences of sleep restriction. *J. Clin. Sleep Med.* **2007**, *3*, 519–528. [CrossRef]
16. Türkarslan, K.K.; Canel Çınarbaş, D. Insomnia Severity Predicts Psychiatric Symptoms: A Cross-Sectional Study Investigating the Partial Mediations of Worry and Rumination. *Psychiatry* **2024**, *87*, 179–193. [CrossRef]
17. Zhang, T.; Xie, X.; Li, Q.; Zhang, L.; Chen, Y.; Ji, G.-J.; Hou, Q.; Li, T.; Zhu, C.; Tian, Y.; et al. Hypogyrification in Generalized Anxiety Disorder and Associated with Insomnia Symptoms. *Nat. Sci. Sleep* **2022**, *14*, 1009–1019. [CrossRef]
18. Giri, P.; Baviskar, M.; Phalke, D. Study of sleep habits and sleep problems among medical students of pravara institute of medical sciences loni, Western maharashtra, India. *Ann. Med. Health Sci. Res.* **2013**, *3*, 51–54. [CrossRef]
19. Nojomi, M.; Ghalhe Bandi, M.F.; Kaffashi, S. Sleep pattern in medical students and residents. *Arch. Iran. Med.* **2009**, *12*, 542–549. [PubMed]
20. Redinger, J.; Kabil, E.; Forkin, K.T.; Kleiman, A.M.; Dunn, L.K. Resting and Recharging: A Narrative Review of Strategies to Improve Sleep During Residency Training. *J. Grad. Med. Educ.* **2022**, *14*, 420–430. [CrossRef] [PubMed]
21. Alshammari, T.; Alseraye, S.; Rogowska, A.; Alrasheed, N.; Alshammari, M. Examining the Indirect Effect of Online Gaming on Depression via Sleep Inequality and Anxiety—A Serial and Parallel Mediation Analysis. *J. Clin. Med.* **2022**, *11*, 7293. [CrossRef] [PubMed]
22. Alshammari, T.; Alseraye, S.; Alqasim, R.; Rogowska, A.; Alrasheed, N.; Alshammari, M. Examining anxiety and stress regarding virtual learning in colleges of health sciences: A cross-sectional study in the era of the COVID-19 pandemic in Saudi Arabia. *Saudi Pharm. J.* **2022**, *30*, 256–264. [CrossRef] [PubMed]
23. Alshammari, T.K.; Alkhodair, A.M.; Alhebshi, H.A.; Rogowska, A.M.; Albaker, A.B.; AL-Damri, N.T.; Bin Dayel, A.F.; Alonazi, A.S.; Alrasheed, N.M.; Alshammari, M.A. Examining Anxiety, Sleep Quality, and Physical Activity as Predictors of Depression among University Students from Saudi Arabia during the Second Wave of the COVID-19 Pandemic. *Int. J. Environ. Res. Public Health* **2022**, *19*, 6262. [CrossRef] [PubMed]
24. Alshammari, T.K.; Rogowska, A.M.; Basharahil, R.F.; Alomar, S.F.; Alseraye, S.S.; Al Juffali, L.A.; Alrasheed, N.M.; Alshammari, M.A. Examining bedtime procrastination, study engagement, and studyholism in undergraduate students, and their association with insomnia. *Front. Psychol.* **2023**, *13*, 1111038. [CrossRef] [PubMed]
25. Byun, J.; Cunningham, S.; Duffy, A.; King, N.; Li, M.; Lindsay, J.A.B.; McGowan, N.M.; Rivera, D.; Saunders, K.E.A. Psychological predictors of insomnia, anxiety and depression in university students: Potential prevention targets. *BJPsych Open* **2022**, *8*, e86. [CrossRef]
26. Al Maqbali, M.; Madkhali, N.; Gleason, A.M.; Dickens, G.L. Fear, stress, anxiety, depression and insomnia related to COVID-19 among undergraduate nursing students: An international survey. *PLoS ONE* **2023**, *18*, e0292470. [CrossRef]
27. Schlarb, A.A.; Friedrich, A.; Claßen, M. Sleep problems in university students—An intervention. *Neuropsychiatr. Dis. Treat.* **2017**, *13*, 1989–2001. [CrossRef]
28. Taylor, D.J.; Bramoweth, A.D.; Grieser, E.A.; Tatum, J.I.; Roane, B.M. Epidemiology of insomnia in college students: Relationship with mental health, quality of life, and substance use difficulties. *Behav. Ther.* **2013**, *44*, 339–348. [CrossRef] [PubMed]
29. Sing, C.Y.; Wong, W.S. Prevalence of insomnia and its psychosocial correlates among college students in Hong Kong. *J. Am. Coll. Health* **2010**, *59*, 174–182. [CrossRef]
30. Abdel-Khalek, A.M. The relation between insomnia and chronic fatigue among a non-clinical sample using questionnaires. *Sleep Hypn.* **2009**, *11*, 9–17.
31. Shibley, H.L.; Malcolm, R.J.; Veatch, L.M. Adolescents with insomnia and substance abuse: Consequences and comorbidities. *J. Psychiatr. Pract.* **2008**, *14*, 146–153. [CrossRef] [PubMed]
32. Grau-López, L.; Grau-López, L.; Daigre, C.; Palma-Álvarez, R.F.; Martínez-Luna, N.; Ros-Cucurull, E.; Ramos-Quiroga, J.A.; Roncero, C. Insomnia Symptoms in Patients with Substance Use Disorders during Detoxification and Associated Clinical Features. *Front. Psychiatry* **2020**, *11*, 540022. [CrossRef] [PubMed]
33. Goodhines, P.A.; Zaso, M.J.; Gellis, L.A.; Park, A. Sleep-related functional impairment as a moderator of risky drinking and subsequent negative drinking consequences in college students. *Addict. Behav.* **2019**, *93*, 146–153. [CrossRef] [PubMed]
34. Vedaa, Ø.; Krossbakken, E.; Grimsrud, I.D.; Bjorvatn, B.; Sivertsen, B.; Magerøy, N.; Einarsen, S.; Pallesen, S. Prospective study of predictors and consequences of insomnia: Personality, lifestyle, mental health, and work-related stressors. *Sleep Med.* **2016**, *20*, 51–58. [CrossRef] [PubMed]
35. Wong, H.Y.; Mo, H.Y.; Potenza, M.N.; Chan, M.N.M.; Lau, W.M.; Chui, T.K.; Pakpour, A.H.; Lin, C.-Y. Relationships between Severity of Internet Gaming Disorder, Severity of Problematic Social Media Use, Sleep Quality and Psychological Distress. *Int. J. Environ. Res. Public Health* **2020**, *17*, 1879. [CrossRef] [PubMed]
36. Shakya, M.; Singh, R.; Chauhan, A.; Rure, D.; Shrivastava, A. Prevalence of internet gaming addiction and its association with sleep quality in medical students. *Ind. Psychiatry J.* **2023**, *32*, S161–S165. [CrossRef] [PubMed]
37. Wong, M.Y.C.; Yuan, G.F.; Liu, C.; Lam, S.K.K.; Fung, H.W. The relationship between internet gaming disorder, sleeping quality, self-compassion, physical activity participation and psychological distress: A path analysis. *Camb. Prism. Glob. Ment. Health* **2024**, *11*, e67. [CrossRef]

38. Fazeli, S.; Mohammadi Zeidi, I.; Lin, C.-Y.; Namdar, P.; Griffiths, M.D.; Ahorsu, D.K.; Pakpour, A.H. Depression, anxiety, and stress mediate the associations between internet gaming disorder, insomnia, and quality of life during the COVID-19 outbreak. *Addict. Behav. Rep.* **2020**, *12*, 100307. [CrossRef] [PubMed]
39. Borsboom, D. A network theory of mental disorders. *World Psychiatry* **2017**, *16*, 5–13. [CrossRef]
40. Fried, E.I.; van Borkulo, C.D.; Epskamp, S. On the Importance of Estimating Parameter Uncertainty in Network Psychometrics: A Response to Forbes et al. (2019). *Multivar. Behav. Res.* **2021**, *56*, 243–248. [CrossRef]
41. Fico, G.; Oliva, V.; De Prisco, M.; Fortea, L.; Fortea, A.; Giménez-Palomo, A.; Anmella, G.; Hidalgo-Mazzei, D.; Vazquez, M.; Gomez-Ramiro, M.; et al. Anxiety and depression played a central role in the COVID-19 mental distress: A network analysis. *J. Affect. Disord.* **2023**, *338*, 384–392. [CrossRef]
42. Peng, P.; Chen, Q.; Liang, M.; Liu, Y.; Chen, S.; Wang, Y.; Yang, Q.; Wang, X.; Li, M.; Wang, Y.; et al. A network analysis of anxiety and depression symptoms among Chinese nurses in the late stage of the COVID-19 pandemic. *Front. Public Health* **2022**, *10*, 996386. [CrossRef]
43. Liu, R.; Chen, X.; Qi, H.; Feng, Y.; Su, Z.; Cheung, T.; Jackson, T.; Lei, H.; Zhang, L.; Xiang, Y.T. Network analysis of depressive and anxiety symptoms in adolescents during and after the COVID-19 outbreak peak. *J. Affect. Disord.* **2022**, *301*, 463–471. [CrossRef]
44. Ramos-Vera, C.; García O'Diana, A.; Basauri-Delgado, M.; Calizaya-Milla, Y.E.; Saintila, J. Network analysis of anxiety and depressive symptoms during the COVID-19 pandemic in older adults in the United Kingdom. *Sci. Rep.* **2024**, *14*, 7741. [CrossRef] [PubMed]
45. Si, T.L.; Chen, P.; Zhang, L.; Sha, S.; Lam, M.I.; Lok, K.-I.; Chow, I.H.I.; Li, J.-X.; Wang, Y.-Y.; Su, Z.; et al. Depression and quality of life among Macau residents in the 2022 COVID-19 pandemic wave from the perspective of network analysis. *Front. Psychol.* **2023**, *14*, 1164232. [CrossRef] [PubMed]
46. Yun, J.Y.; Myung, S.J.; Kim, K.S. Associations among the workplace violence, burnout, depressive symptoms, suicidality, and turnover intention in training physicians: A network analysis of nationwide survey. *Sci. Rep.* **2023**, *13*, 16804. [CrossRef] [PubMed]
47. Levinson, C.A.; Cusack, C.; Brown, M.L.; Smith, A.R. A network approach can improve eating disorder conceptualization and treatment. *Nat. Rev. Psychol.* **2022**, *1*, 419–430. [CrossRef]
48. Peng, P.; Liang, M.; Wang, Q.; Lu, L.; Wu, Q.; Chen, Q. Night shifts, insomnia, anxiety, and depression among Chinese nurses during the COVID-19 pandemic remission period: A network approach. *Front. Public Health* **2022**, *10*, 1040298. [CrossRef]
49. Cai, H.; Zhao, Y.-j.; Xing, X.; Tian, T.; Qian, W.; Liang, S.; Wang, Z.; Cheung, T.; Su, Z.; Tang, Y.-L.; et al. Network Analysis of Comorbid Anxiety and Insomnia among Clinicians with Depressive Symptoms during the Late Stage of the COVID-19 Pandemic: A Cross-Sectional Study. *Nat. Sci. Sleep* **2022**, *14*, 1351–1362. [CrossRef]
50. Li, J.; Luo, C.; Liu, L.; Huang, A.; Ma, Z.; Chen, Y.; Deng, Y.; Zhao, J. Depression, anxiety, and insomnia symptoms among Chinese college students: A network analysis across pandemic stages. *J. Affect. Disord.* **2024**, *356*, 54–63. [CrossRef]
51. Parkes, J.D. The culture of insomnia. *Brain* **2009**, *132*, 3488–3493. [CrossRef]
52. Whitehead, K.; Beaumont, M. Insomnia: A cultural history. *Lancet* **2018**, *391*, 2408–2409. [CrossRef] [PubMed]
53. Mokyr, J.; Vickers, C.; Ziebarth, N.L. The History of Technological Anxiety and the Future of Economic Growth: Is This Time Different? *J. Econ. Perspect.* **2015**, *29*, 31–50. [CrossRef]
54. Hofmann, S.G. Cognitive factors that maintain social anxiety disorder: A comprehensive model and its treatment implications. *Cogn. Behav. Ther.* **2007**, *36*, 193–209. [CrossRef] [PubMed]
55. Knutson, K.L. Sociodemographic and cultural determinants of sleep deficiency: Implications for cardiometabolic disease risk. *Soc. Sci. Med.* **2013**, *79*, 7–15. [CrossRef] [PubMed]
56. Johnson, S.U.; Ulvenes, P.G.; Øktedalen, T.; Hoffart, A. Psychometric Properties of the General Anxiety Disorder 7-Item (GAD-7) Scale in a Heterogeneous Psychiatric Sample. *Front. Psychol.* **2019**, *10*, 1713. [CrossRef]
57. Spitzer, R.L.; Kroenke, K.; Williams, J.B.; Löwe, B. A brief measure for assessing generalized anxiety disorder: The GAD-7. *Arch. Intern. Med.* **2006**, *166*, 1092–1097. [CrossRef] [PubMed]
58. Sawaya, H.; Atoui, M.; Hamadeh, A.; Zeinoun, P.; Nahas, Z. Adaptation and initial validation of the Patient Health Questionnaire–9 (PHQ-9) and the Generalized Anxiety Disorder–7 Questionnaire (GAD-7) in an Arabic speaking Lebanese psychiatric outpatient sample. *Psychiatry Res.* **2016**, *239*, 245–252. [CrossRef] [PubMed]
59. Soldatos, C.R.; Dikeos, D.G.; Paparrigopoulos, T.J. Athens Insomnia Scale: Validation of an instrument based on ICD-10 criteria. *J. Psychosom. Res.* **2000**, *48*, 555–560. [CrossRef] [PubMed]
60. Jahrami, H.; Trabelsi, K.; Saif, Z.; Manzar, M.D.; BaHammam, A.S.; Vitiello, M.V. Reliability generalization meta-analysis of the Athens Insomnia Scale and its translations: Examining internal consistency and test-retest validity. *Sleep Med.* **2023**, *111*, 133–145. [CrossRef]
61. Hallit, S.; Haddad, C.; Hallit, R.; Al Karaki, G.; Malaeb, D.; Sacre, H.; Kheir, N.; Hajj, A.; Salameh, P. Validation of selected sleeping disorders related scales in Arabic among the Lebanese Population. *Sleep Biol. Rhythm.* **2019**, *17*, 183–189. [CrossRef]
62. Pontes, H.M.; Griffiths, M.D. Measuring DSM-5 internet gaming disorder: Development and validation of a short psychometric scale. *Comput. Hum. Behav.* **2015**, *45*, 137–143. [CrossRef]

63. Gomez, R.; Stavropoulos, V.; Beard, C.; Pontes, H.M. Item Response Theory Analysis of the Recoded Internet Gaming Disorder Scale-Short-Form (IGDS9-SF). *Int. J. Ment. Health Addict.* **2019**, *17*, 859–879. [CrossRef]
64. Poon, L.Y.; Tsang, H.W.; Chan, T.Y.; Man, S.W.; Ng, L.Y.; Wong, Y.L.; Lin, C.-Y.; Chien, C.-W.; Griffiths, M.D.; Pontes, H.M. Psychometric properties of the internet gaming disorder scale–short-form (IGDS9-SF): Systematic review. *J. Med. Internet Res.* **2021**, *23*, e26821. [CrossRef]
65. Pontes, H.M.; Stavropoulos, V.; Griffiths, M.D. Measurement Invariance of the Internet Gaming Disorder Scale–Short-Form (IGDS9-SF) between the United States of America, India and the United Kingdom. *Psychiatry Res.* **2017**, *257*, 472–478. [CrossRef] [PubMed]
66. Baiumy, S.; Elella, E.A.; Hewedi, D.; Elkholy, H. Internet gaming disorder scale: Arabic version validation. *Middle East. Curr. Psychiatry* **2018**, *25*, 13–15. [CrossRef]
67. National Institute of Mental Health (NIMH). Any Anxiety Disorder. Available online: https://www.nimh.nih.gov/health/statistics/any-anxiety-disorder (accessed on 24 June 2024).
68. Appleton, S.L.; Reynolds, A.C.; Gill, T.K.; Melaku, Y.A.; Adams, R.J. Insomnia Prevalence Varies with Symptom Criteria Used with Implications for Epidemiological Studies: Role of Anthropometrics, Sleep Habit, and Comorbidities. *Nat. Sci. Sleep* **2022**, *14*, 775–790. [CrossRef]
69. Perlis, M.L.; Vargas, I.; Ellis, J.G.; Grandner, M.A.; Morales, K.H.; Gencarelli, A.; Khader, W.; Kloss, J.D.; Gooneratne, N.S.; Thase, M.E. The Natural History of Insomnia: The incidence of acute insomnia and subsequent progression to chronic insomnia or recovery in good sleeper subjects. *Sleep* **2020**, *43*, zsz299. [CrossRef] [PubMed]
70. Stevens, M.W.; Dorstyn, D.; Delfabbro, P.H.; King, D.L. Global prevalence of gaming disorder: A systematic review and meta-analysis. *Aust. N. Z. J. Psychiatry* **2021**, *55*, 553–568. [CrossRef]
71. Dragioti, E.; Levin, L.-Å.; Bernfort, L.; Larsson, B.; Gerdle, B. Insomnia severity and its relationship with demographics, pain features, anxiety, and depression in older adults with and without pain: Cross-sectional population-based results from the PainS65+ cohort. *Ann. Gen. Psychiatry* **2017**, *16*, 15. [CrossRef]
72. Li, Y.I.; Starr, L.R.; Wray-Lake, L. Insomnia mediates the longitudinal relationship between anxiety and depressive symptoms in a nationally representative sample of adolescents. *Depress. Anxiety* **2018**, *35*, 583–591. [CrossRef] [PubMed]
73. Prather, A.A.; Vogelzangs, N.; Penninx, B.W. Sleep duration, insomnia, and markers of systemic inflammation: Results from the Netherlands Study of Depression and Anxiety (NESDA). *J. Psychiatr. Res.* **2015**, *60*, 95–102. [CrossRef]
74. Vollrath, M.; Wicki, W.; Angst, J. The Zurich study. *Eur. Arch. Psychiatry Neurol. Sci.* **1989**, *239*, 113–124. [CrossRef]
75. Li, C.; Xia, L.; Ma, J.; Li, S.; Liang, S.; Ma, X.; Wang, T.; Li, M.; Wen, H.; Jiang, G. Dynamic functional abnormalities in generalized anxiety disorders and their increased network segregation of a hyperarousal brain state modulated by insomnia. *J. Affect. Disord.* **2019**, *246*, 338–345. [CrossRef] [PubMed]
76. Huang, Z.; Liang, P.; Jia, X.; Zhan, S.; Li, N.; Ding, Y.; Lu, J.; Wang, Y.; Li, K. Abnormal amygdala connectivity in patients with primary insomnia: Evidence from resting state fMRI. *Eur. J. Radiol.* **2012**, *81*, 1288–1295. [CrossRef]
77. Šimić, G.; Tkalčić, M.; Vukić, V.; Mulc, D.; Španić, E.; Šagud, M.; Olucha-Bordonau, F.E.; Vukšić, M.; Hof, P.R. Understanding Emotions: Origins and Roles of the Amygdala. *Biomolecules* **2021**, *11*, 823. [CrossRef] [PubMed]
78. Chowdhury, A.I.; Ghosh, S.; Hasan, M.F.; Khandakar, K.A.S.; Azad, F. Prevalence of insomnia among university students in South Asian Region: A systematic review of studies. *J. Prev. Med. Hyg.* **2020**, *61*, E525.
79. Mbous, Y.P.V.; Nili, M.; Mohamed, R.; Dwibedi, N. Psychosocial Correlates of Insomnia Among College Students. *Prev. Chronic Dis.* **2022**, *19*, E60. [CrossRef]
80. Amaral, M.O.P.; de Figueiredo Pereira, C.M.; Martins, D.I.S.; de Serpa, C.d.R.D.N.; Sakellarides, C.T. Prevalence and risk factors for insomnia among Portuguese adolescents. *Eur. J. Pediatr.* **2013**, *172*, 1305–1311. [CrossRef]
81. Buysse, D.J.; Angst, J.; Gamma, A.; Ajdacic, V.; Eich, D.; Rössler, W. Prevalence, Course, and Comorbidity of Insomnia and Depression in Young Adults. *Sleep* **2008**, *31*, 473–480. [CrossRef]
82. Almohammadi, A.L.; Alghamdi, M.; Almohammadi, E.L. Socio-demographic and Lifestyle Determinants of Insomnia among Adult Patients Attending Primary Healthcare Centres, Jeddah: A Cross-sectional Study. *J. Clin. Diagn. Res.* **2019**, *13*, LC14–LC20. [CrossRef]
83. Glasbeek, M.P.; Inhulsen, M.-B.M.R.; Busch, V.; van Stralen, M.M. Sleep reduction in adolescents: Socio-demographic factors and the mediating role of sleep hygiene practices. *Sleep Epidemiol.* **2022**, *2*, 100024. [CrossRef]
84. Alfawaz, H.A.; Khan, N.; Yakout, S.M.; Khattak, M.N.K.; Alsaikhan, A.A.; Almousa, A.A.; Alsuwailem, T.A.; Almjlad, T.M.; Alamri, N.A.; Alshammari, S.G.; et al. Prevalence, Predictors, and Awareness of Coffee Consumption and Its Trend among Saudi Female Students. *Int. J. Environ. Res. Public Health* **2020**, *17*, 20. [CrossRef] [PubMed]
85. Eltyeb, E.E.; Al-Makramani, A.A.; Mustafa, M.M.; Shubayli, S.M.; Madkhali, K.A.; Zaalah, S.A.; Ghalibi, A.T.; Ali, S.A.; Ibrahim, A.M.; Basheer, R.A. Caffeine Consumption and Its Potential Health Effects on Saudi Adolescents in Jazan. *Cureus* **2023**, *15*, e44091. [CrossRef] [PubMed]
86. Things to Do in Saudi After Dark. Available online: https://www.sotc.in/blog/destinations/international/dubai-holidays/things-to-do-in-saudi-after-dark (accessed on 24 June 2024).

87. Kupfer, D.; Foster, F.G. Interval between onset of sleep and rapid-eye-movement sleep as an indicator of depression. *Lancet* **1972**, *300*, 684–686. [CrossRef] [PubMed]
88. Spiegelhalder, K.; Scholtes, C.; Riemann, D. The association between insomnia and cardiovascular diseases. *Nat. Sci. Sleep* **2010**, *2*, 71–78. [CrossRef]
89. Duraccio, K.M.; Simmons, D.M.; Beebe, D.W.; Byars, K.C. Relationship of overweight and obesity to insomnia severity, sleep quality, and insomnia improvement in a clinically referred pediatric sample. *J. Clin. Sleep Med.* **2022**, *18*, 1083–1091. [CrossRef] [PubMed]
90. Beydoun, H.A.; Beydoun, M.A.; Weiss, J.; Hossain, S.; Huang, S.; Alemu, B.T.; Zonderman, A.B. Insomnia as a predictor of diagnosed memory problems: 2006–2016 Health and Retirement Study. *Sleep Med.* **2021**, *80*, 158–166. [CrossRef] [PubMed]
91. Dong, Y.; Yang, F.M. Insomnia symptoms predict both future hypertension and depression. *Prev. Med.* **2019**, *123*, 41–47. [CrossRef]
92. Kupfer, D.J. REM latency: A psychobiologic marker for primary depressive disease. *Biol. Psychiatry* **1976**, *11*, 159–174.
93. Hein, M.; Lanquart, J.-P.; Loas, G.; Hubain, P.; Linkowski, P. Prevalence and risk factors of type 2 diabetes in insomnia sufferers: A study on 1311 individuals referred for sleep examinations. *Sleep Med.* **2018**, *46*, 37–45. [CrossRef] [PubMed]
94. Bocci Benucci, S.; Tonini, B.; Casale, S.; Fioravanti, G. Testing the role of extended thinking in predicting craving and problematic social network sites use. *Addict. Behav.* **2024**, *155*, 108042. [CrossRef] [PubMed]
95. World Health Organization. *Classification of Mental and Behavioural Disorders: Clinical Descriptions and Diagnostic Guidelines*; World Health Organization: Geneva, Switzerland, 2019.
96. Ebner, K.; Soucek, R.; Selenko, E. Perceived quality of internships and employability perceptions: The mediating role of career-entry worries. *Educ. Train.* **2021**, *63*, 579–596. [CrossRef]
97. Bard, H.A.; O'Driscoll, C.; Miller, C.B.; Henry, A.L.; Cape, J.; Espie, C.A. Insomnia, depression, and anxiety symptoms interact and individually impact functioning: A network and relative importance analysis in the context of insomnia. *Sleep Med.* **2023**, *101*, 505–514. [CrossRef] [PubMed]
98. Frøjd, L.A.; Papageorgiou, C.; Munkhaugen, J.; Moum, T.; Sverre, E.; Nordhus, I.H.; Dammen, T. Worry and rumination predict insomnia in patients with coronary heart disease: A cross-sectional study with long-term follow-up. *J. Clin. Sleep Med.* **2022**, *18*, 779–787. [CrossRef] [PubMed]
99. Marchica, L.A.; Mills, D.J.; Derevensky, J.L.; Montreuil, T.C. The Role of Emotion Regulation in Video Gaming and Gambling Disorder: A Systematic Review. *Can. J. Addict.* **2019**, *10*, 19–29. [CrossRef]
100. Hariwijaksono, H. The Length of Time Children Play Emotional Reaction Games (9–11 Years). *Health Res. J.* **2024**, *1*, 192–197.
101. Xu, J.M. *Understanding Motivational Factors of Problematic Video Gaming in the USMC and USN*; Naval Postgraduate School, Defense Technical Information Center (DTIC): Monterey, CA, USA, 2022.
102. Blanken, T.F.; Van Der Zweerde, T.; Van Straten, A.; Van Someren, E.J.W.; Borsboom, D.; Lancee, J. Introducing Network Intervention Analysis to Investigate Sequential, Symptom-Specific Treatment Effects: A Demonstration in Co-Occurring Insomnia and Depression. *Psychother. Psychosom.* **2019**, *88*, 52–54. [CrossRef] [PubMed]
103. Santos, H., Jr.; Fried, E.I.; Asafu-Adjei, J.; Ruiz, R.J. Network Structure of Perinatal Depressive Symptoms in Latinas: Relationship to Stress and Reproductive Biomarkers. *Res. Nurs. Health* **2017**, *40*, 218–228. [CrossRef]
104. Khodarahimi, S.; Pole, N. Cognitive Behavior Therapy and Worry Reduction in an Outpatient with Generalized Anxiety Disorder. *Clin. Case Stud.* **2010**, *9*, 53–62. [CrossRef]
105. Ladouceur, R.; Dugas, M.J.; Freeston, M.H.; Léger, E.; Gagnon, F.; Thibodeau, N. Efficacy of a cognitive–behavioral treatment for generalized anxiety disorder: Evaluation in a controlled clinical trial. *J. Consult. Clin. Psychol.* **2000**, *68*, 957–964. [CrossRef] [PubMed]
106. Renna, M.E.; Quintero, J.M.; Soffer, A.; Pino, M.; Ader, L.; Fresco, D.M.; Mennin, D.S. A pilot study of emotion regulation therapy for generalized anxiety and depression: Findings from a diverse sample of young adults. *Behav. Ther.* **2018**, *49*, 403–418. [CrossRef] [PubMed]
107. Brandeis University. Brandeis Counseling Center. Available online: https://www.brandeis.edu/counseling/services-programs/cbt-program.html (accessed on 20 June 2024).
108. Young, J.F.; Mufson, L.; Gallop, R. Preventing depression: A randomized trial of interpersonal psychotherapy-adolescent skills training. *Depress. Anxiety* **2010**, *27*, 426–433. [CrossRef] [PubMed]
109. Stice, E.; Burton, E.; Bearman, S.K.; Rohde, P. Randomized trial of a brief depression prevention program: An elusive search for a psychosocial placebo control condition. *Behav. Res. Ther.* **2007**, *45*, 863–876. [CrossRef] [PubMed]
110. Primavera, D.; Aviles Gonzalez, C.I.; Romano, F.; Kalcev, G.; Pinna, S.; Minerba, L.; Scano, A.; Orrù, G.; Cossu, G. Does the Response to a Stressful Condition in Older Adults with Life Rhythm Dysregulations Provide Evidence of the Existence of the "Dysregulation of Mood, Energy, and Social Rhythms Syndrome"? *Healthcare* **2024**, *12*, 87. [CrossRef] [PubMed]
111. Primavera, D.; Cossu, G.; Marchegiani, S.; Preti, A.; Nardi, A.E. Does the Dysregulation of Social Rhythms Syndrome (DYMERS) be Considered an Essential Component of Panic Disorders? *Clin. Pract. Epidemiol. Ment. Health* **2024**, *20*, e17450179293272. [CrossRef] [PubMed]
112. Akiskal, H.S. The emergence of the bipolar spectrum: Validation along clinical-epidemiologic and familial-genetic lines. *Psychopharmacol. Bull.* **2007**, *40*, 99–115. [PubMed]

113. Carta, M.G.; Fornaro, M.; Primavera, D.; Nardi, A.E.; Karam, E. Dysregulation of mood, energy, and social rhythms syndrome (DYMERS): A working hypothesis. *J. Public Health Res.* **2024**, *13*, 22799036241248022. [CrossRef]
114. Epskamp, S.; Borsboom, D.; Fried, E.I. Estimating psychological networks and their accuracy: A tutorial paper. *Behav. Res. Methods* **2018**, *50*, 195–212. [CrossRef]

Disclaimer/Publisher's Note: The statements, opinions and data contained in all publications are solely those of the individual author(s) and contributor(s) and not of MDPI and/or the editor(s). MDPI and/or the editor(s) disclaim responsibility for any injury to people or property resulting from any ideas, methods, instructions or products referred to in the content.

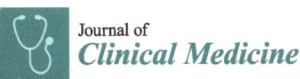

Article

The Relevance of Insomnia Among Healthcare Workers: A Post-Pandemic COVID-19 Analysis

Carlos Roncero [1,2,3,4,*], José Bravo-Grande [2,5], Diego Remón-Gallo [2,3,4], Pilar Andrés-Olivera [2,3,6], Candela Payo-Rodríguez [6], Alicia Fernández-Parra [1], Lourdes Aguilar [2,3,4,6], Marta Peña [1] and Armando González-Sánchez [2,4,7,*]

[1] Health Science Faculty, Miguel de Cervantes European University (UEMC), Valladolid (Spain). C. del Padre Julio Chevalier, 2, 47012 Valladolid, Spain; afernandezp@uemc.es (A.F.-P.)
[2] Instituto de Investigación Biomédica de Salamanca (IBSAL), Hospital Virgen de la Vega, 10 ª Planta, Paseo de San Vicente, 58-182, 37007 Salamanca, Spain; jlbravo@saludcastillayleon.es (J.B.-G.); d.remon@usal.es (D.R.-G.); mpolivera@saludcastillayleon.es (P.A.-O.); lourdesaguilar@usal.es (L.A.)
[3] Psychiatric Unit, School of Medicine, University of Salamanca (Spain), Campus Miguel de Unamuno, Calle Alfonso X El Sabio s/n, 37007 Salamanca, Spain
[4] Network of Research in Primary Care of Addictions (RIAPAD), Instituto Carlos III (Spain), 28029 Madrid, Spain
[5] Department of Occupational Health—Prevention of Occupational Risks, Salamanca Health Area & University of Salamanca Health Care Complex, Paseo de San Vicente 58-182, 37007 Salamanca, Spain
[6] Psychiatry Service, University of Salamanca Health Care Complex, Paseo de San Vicente 58-182, 37007 Salamanca, Spain; cpayo@saludcastillayleon.es
[7] Facultad de Psicología, Universidad Pontificia de Salamanca (UPSA), C/Compañía, 5, 37002 Salamanca, Spain
* Correspondence: drcarlosroncero@gmail.com (C.R.); armando_gonzalez@usal.es (A.G.-S.)

Abstract: Background: Insomnia significantly impairs healthcare worker (HCW) well-being, particularly amid COVID-19 sequelae and shift work demands. We aimed to assess the prevalence of insomnia among HCWs, identify those needing clinical intervention, analyze shift work as a potential risk factor, and explore associations with COVID-19 sequelae and psychiatric comorbidities. **Methods:** A cross-sectional online survey was administered at the University of Salamanca University Care Complex (CAUSA) from March 2023 to January 2024. Validated scales (Insomnia Severity Index, Patient Health Questionnaire-4, Generalized Anxiety Disorder Scale-2) were used to measure insomnia, depression, and anxiety. Participants scoring ISI ≥ 7 were invited for Occupational Medicine follow-up. Descriptive and inferential analyses were performed. **Results:** Overall, 1121 HCWs participated (mean age 44.59 ± 11.78, 78.3% women). The mean ISI score was 10.5 ± 5.8 (subclinical insomnia), with 22.7% reporting moderate and 3% reporting severe insomnia. Depression and anxiety affected 28.4% and 33% of respondents, respectively. Shift workers had poorer sleep (mean ISI 11.3 ± 0.9 vs. 8.8 ± 0.3, $p < 0.001$). Individuals reporting COVID-19 sequelae were 3.1 times more likely to have insomnia than those who did not (mean ISI 13.89 ± 5.9 vs. 10.33 ± 5.7, $p < 0.001$). Over one-quarter reported at least the monthly use of sleep or psychiatric medications. **Conclusions:** Insomnia remains prevalent among HCWs, influenced by shift work, COVID-19 sequelae, and mental health factors. Targeted, multidisciplinary interventions, e.g., workplace policy changes, mental health programs, and shift schedule adjustments are urgently needed to safeguard well-being, reduce burnout, and maintain quality patient care. Ensuring adequate sleep is central to minimizing errors and preserving professional performance. Future studies should investigate the impact of coordinated workplace strategies to effectively address insomnia.

Keywords: insomnia; mental health impact; shift work; occupational hazard; anxiety; depression; COVID-19 sequelae; multidisciplinary intervention; quality of care; sleep disorders

1. Introduction

Sleep disturbances such as insomnia, sleep apnea, and circadian rhythm disorders are considered a public health epidemic [1]. They are common in healthcare workers (HCWs), who frequently face clinical situations with a high emotional burden and can perpetuate the high rates of associated burnout [2]. Insomnia can lead to significant morbidity and exacerbate medical and psychiatric conditions. Moreover, poor sleep, whether in quantity or quality, increases the risk of premature aging, obesity, and cardiovascular diseases [3,4].

Insomnia comprises daytime and nighttime symptoms that seriously affect quality of life and well-being. It is characterized by difficulty falling asleep or by fatigue or dysfunction during the day [4,5]. HCWs often exhibit a high prevalence of insomnia, with aggravating factors such as shift work [6]. In addition, the coexistence of insomnia and mental illness is common. In a systematic review and meta-analysis on the prevalence of depression, anxiety, and insomnia among HCWs during the COVID-19 pandemic (n = 33,062) [7], the prevalence of insomnia was estimated at 38.9%. The authors also found a pooled prevalence of anxiety and depression of 23.2% and 22.8%, respectively. As shown by studies performed on HCWs worldwide, including Spain, this scenario was aggravated after the pandemic [8–16] and requires specific measures to prevent it from becoming chronic.

This study is part of a more ambitious study. Because worrying levels of sleep problems were detected among the working population of the University of Salamanca Health Care Complex (known by its Spanish acronym CAUSA), it was decided to extend this screening to the whole workforce of the hospital. So, the aim was to first detect the workers affected by sleep problems and who wanted specific treatment. Subsequently, and with the people detected, these data would be provided to the occupational medicine unit, so that they could offer them group treatment and continue to evaluate them. Occupational medicine would then refer the HCWs who were particularly affected and who wanted it to the mental health unit for specialized treatment using both psychological and pharmacological therapy.

In view of these data, the Services of Psychiatry and Occupational Health of CAUSA carried out a study on the sleep disturbances experienced by the HCWs of this center after the COVID-19 pandemic. The objectives were as follows: (1) to evaluate the prevalence of insomnia among HCWs; (2) to identify individuals with insomnia who could be referred to the Occupational Medicine Service to undergo interventions to improve sleep quality; (3) to characterize the job profiles most affected by insomnia; (4) to analyze the relationship between sleep problems and the consequences of COVID-19; (5) to evaluate psychiatric comorbidities and their pharmacological treatment; and (6) to evaluate the presence of depression and anxiety.

2. Materials and Methods

A cross-sectional study was carried out through a survey completed by HCWs of CAUSA. An online questionnaire was designed (see Appendix S1) and made available via the CAUSA intranet. The HCWs were invited to participate in the study through posters on the walls (see the Supplementary Files) and advertisements on the institution's website, and emails were sent to all HCWs from Human Resources, inviting them to participate in the survey. Participants completed the questionnaire between 7 March 2023 and 5 January 2024.

The questionnaire consisted of 70 questions grouped into 8 blocks and had an estimated response time of 15 min. It included 11 sociodemographic questions referring to the job position, 22 about protective or risk factors for sleep quality and the consequences of poor sleep quality, and 10 about the consumption of related medications/substances. As for the work modalities, 2 types of shifts were considered, namely shifts of 7-7-10 h (morning 8:00 am–3:00 pm, afternoon 3:00 pm–10:00 pm, and night 10:00 pm–8:00 am) and shifts of 12 h.

Sleep quality and its consequences were assessed using three validated scales with good psychometric properties (Table 1). The Insomnia Severity Index (ISI) [17–19] was used to evaluate sleep quality. The scale has a total score range of 0–28, where 0–7 indicates the absence of clinical insomnia, 8–14 indicates subclinical insomnia, 15–21 indicates moderate clinical insomnia, and 22–28 indicates severe clinical insomnia. The Patient Health Questionnaire-4 (PHQ-4) [20,21] is a self-administered tool used for evaluating mental health in the population. It consists of the PHQ-2 [22,23], a shortened version of the PHQ-9 [24] for depression, and the GAD-2 [25], derived from the GAD-7 [26] for anxiety. By combining these two components, the PHQ-4 provides a concise four-item measure that assesses both depression and anxiety.

Table 1. Scales included in the questionnaire.

Scale	Parameters	Psychometric Properties
Insomnia Severity Index (ISI) [8,17–19]	Impact on quality of life	$\alpha = 0.82$. Correlation: 0.35 for insomnia; 0.56 for impact of insomnia; 0.50 for dissatisfaction with sleep.
Patient Health Questionnaire (PHQ-4) [20,21,27]	Depression and anxiety	$\alpha > 0.8$; $r = 0.2$ with Study Short Form-20.
Patient Health Questionnaire (PHQ-2) [22,23,26]	Major depressive disorder	The optimal PHQ-2 cut-off score was 3, achieved with a sensitivity of 74.6% and specificity of 93.9%. Area under the curve: 0.92 (CI 0.91–0.93).
Generalized Anxiety Disorder Scale-2 Questionnaire (GAD-2) [26]	Generalized anxiety disorder	Both the GAD-7 scale and its 2 core items (GAD-2) performed well (area under the curve, 0.80 to 0.91) as screening tools for anxiety disorders.

At the end of the questionnaire, an option was enabled for participants with scores greater than 7 points on the ISI (corresponding to at least subclinical insomnia) to provide an email address or telephone number so that the Occupational Medicine Service could contact them to offer strategies for treating sleep problems. Although anonymity was broken, this circumstance was recorded in the protocol.

Participants were asked whether they had received a formal diagnosis of any pathology from a qualified healthcare professional.

In this study, missing data were handled by excluding participants from specific analyses if they lacked data on the variable(s) of interest. Consequently, the sample size differs across analyses. Prior to conducting the main analyses, we performed preliminary checks for patterns in missing responses; no systematic or non-random patterns were detected, suggesting that the missing data mechanism did not introduce bias in the results.

A descriptive analysis of the data was performed. Frequencies, percentages, means with their standard deviation (SD), and Mann–Whitney U, Kruskal–Wallis K, Spearman rho, and Chi-Square tests were used. A confidence level of 5% was established. Data were analyzed using SPSS, Version 28.0 [28].

This study was performed in accordance with the Declaration of Helsinki on medical research in human beings in its latest version and with the applicable regulations on Good

Clinical Practice. The confidentiality of the participants' personal data was preserved in accordance with Organic Law 3/2018, of December 5, on the Protection of Personal Data and guarantee of digital rights. Informed consent was obtained from each participant. This study was approved on 24 October 2022 by the local bioethics committee of CAUSA together with the Ethics Committee for Drug Research of the Salamanca Health Area (code PI 2002101152).

3. Results

3.1. Sample

A total of 1121 questionnaires were completed, representing around 30.6% of all HCWs (see the calculation of the sample size in the supplementary files). In total, 61 percent of the questionnaires were answered completely and 39% partially. The characteristics of the study sample are described in Table 2.

Table 2. Characteristics of the study sample.

Characteristic	Values	IC95%
Age, years (mean ± SD)	44.59 ± 11.78	
Sex (n, %)		
Women	760 (78.3)	10.31–11.16
Men	211 (21.7)	8.81–10.57
Work modality (n, %)		
Bachelor's degree	700 (72.2)	
Permanent contract	309 (31.9)	
Temporary contract	191 (19.7)	
Job category * (n, %)		
A2	304 (31.4)	
A1	198 (20.4)	
C1-C2	195 (20.1)	
Overtime in the previous month (n, %)	307 (31.6)	
Extra hours paid	67 (21.8)	
Shift work (n, %)	647 (57.7)	
7-7-10 h schedule	542 (83.7)	10.84–11.83
12 h schedule	45 (6.9)	9.51–13.15
Both (in the last month)	59 (9.2)	9.26–12.6
Including nights	394 (51.4)	
Rotating shift	364 (47.5)	
Work during COVID-19 (n, %)	598 (78)	
COVID-19 sequelae (n, %)	100 (13)	

* A2: nurses, occupational therapists, nutrition graduates, and speech therapists; A1: graduate specialists; C1–C2: senior technicians, auxiliary care technicians, and pharmacy technicians.

Of the respondents, 26.4% (n = 297) filled out the telephone and/or email fields to be contacted by the Occupational Medicine Service.

3.2. Sleep Characteristics

The mean score on the ISI scale (n = 915) was 10.51 ± 5.8, corresponding to subclinical insomnia. Moderate clinical insomnia was present in 22.7% (n = 208) and severe clinical insomnia in 3% (n = 27) (Figure 1). In a total of 24 (3.1%) participants, the characteristics of a severe sleep disorder were detected.

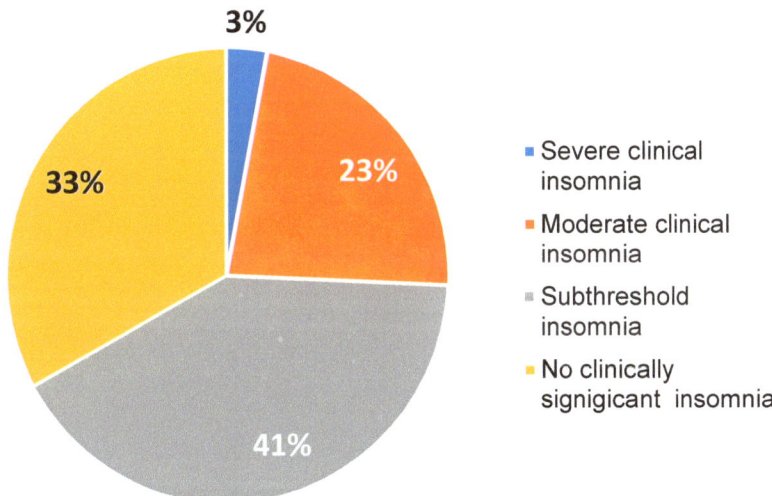

Figure 1. Pie chart of Insomnia Severity Index scores obtained of the sample during the study (n = 915).

Poorer sleep quality was observed in women, who obtained an average ISI score of 10.74 ± 0.2 (compared to 9.69 ± 0.4 for men), although the differences were not statistically significant ($p = 0.325$). ISI scores were positively correlated with age (correlation coefficient, $r = 0.086$; $p = 0.010$).

3.3. Interaction Between Work and Sleep

Participants who worked shifts had poorer sleep quality than those on a continuous schedule. Specifically, the 7-7-10 h shift group had a mean ISI of 11.3 ± 0.2 ($p < 0.001$ vs. continuous schedule), the 12-h shift group had 11.3 ± 0.9 ($p = 0.016$), and the group working both shifts had 10.93 ± 0.8 ($p = 0.012$), whereas participants on a continuous schedule had 8.8 ± 0.3 (Figure 2). The differences were significant between participants who did not work shifts and those who worked 7-7-10h shifts ($p < 0.001$). However, no significant differences were found between the rest of the groups.

Nine participants (1.2%) had missed work in the previous month owing to poor sleep quality (n = 766).

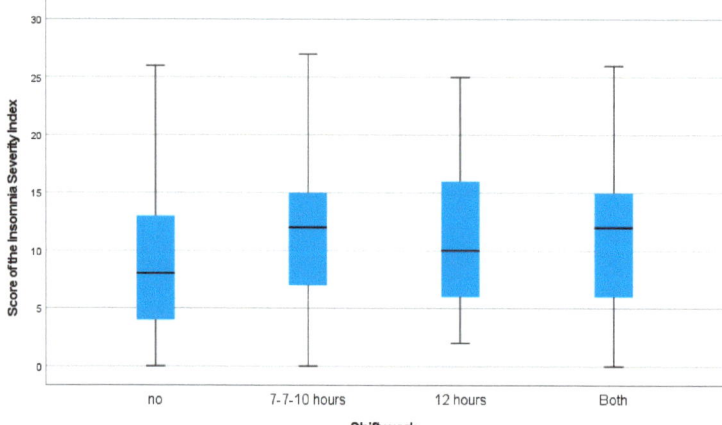

Figure 2. Boxplot of Insomnia Severity Index scores obtained during the study according to work schedule (n = 915).

3.4. Interaction Between COVID-19 and Sleep

COVID-19 sequelae were reported by 13.0% (n = 100) of participants, and this was a determining factor in poor sleep quality ($p = 0.003$). The odds ratio showed that the probability of sleep disturbances was 3.1 times higher in participants with COVID-19 sequelae than in those without (mean ISI scores 13.89 ± 5.9 vs. 10.33 ± 5.7, respectively), which was statistically significant ($p < 0.001$). No significant differences in the ISI scores were found between those who worked or did not work during the first waves of the COVID-19 pandemic ($p = 0.209$).

3.5. Psychiatric Comorbidities

Of those who completed the mental health questionnaires (n = 799), 28.4% (n = 226) had major depressive disorder and 33% (n = 264) had generalized anxiety disorder.

Of these, 94 were currently undergoing psychological or psychiatric treatment. Concurrent cases of depression and generalized anxiety disorder were observed in 166 individuals (20.8%).

Medication Consumption

Among the participants, 15.5% and 23.3% reported taking medications at least once a month to treat depression/anxiety or to fall asleep, respectively. Of the latter, 27.6% (n = 51) did so without a medical prescription; 8 participants reported using illegal drugs (cannabinoids, n = 6; stimulants and depressants, n = 1; stimulants, depressants, and cannabis, n = 1).

4. Discussion

This real-world study showed that sleep disorders, mainly insomnia, are highly prevalent among HCWs (25.7% for severe and moderate insomnia) and that shift work and the sequelae of COVID-19 may act as aggravating factors. Consequently, a significant proportion of workers face sleep problems that can affect their work performance and personal well-being. Remarkably, only 3.1% of the participants were currently diagnosed with a sleep disorder, and more than 26% of the respondents agreed to be contacted by the Occupational Medicine Service for assistance to solve their sleep problems.

4.1. Interaction Between COVID-19 and Sleep

We confirm that the sleep of HCWs was particularly affected by the COVID-19 pandemic and that these individuals were exposed to more stressful circumstances than other professionals. A systematic review and meta-analysis estimated the prevalence of insomnia symptoms in HCWs to be nearly 40% during the COVID-19 pandemic [7]. A 2021 meta-analysis of COVID-19-related stress and psychiatric symptoms in nurses (93 studies encompassing 93,112 nurses) [29] showed that over one-third reported stress, sleep disorders, and increased anxiety symptoms. The pooled prevalence of insomnia was 43% [29]. Furthermore, in a Spanish cohort of HCWs analyzed in April 2020 (n = 1422), over half reported symptoms of post-traumatic stress and anxiety disorders, and nearly 50% had experienced symptoms of depression, with women and younger individuals showing a higher risk [30]. Being a woman and working 12 h or 24 h shifts were risk factors for anxiety and depression. In our study, poorer sleep quality was observed in women and older individuals, although the differences were not statistically significant.

The probability of insomnia was 3.1 times higher in HCWs with COVID-19 sequelae, this difference being significant. Major depressive and generalized anxiety disorders were present in 28.4% and 33% of the samples, respectively, consistent with the frequently reported coexistence of insomnia and anxiety/depression [31]. In Spain, a meta-analysis of more than 82,000 individuals showed a pooled prevalence of anxiety symptoms and depression of 20% and 22%, respectively, during the COVID-19 pandemic; that of insomnia was 57% [32]. In another meta-analysis of studies comprising 271 Spanish HCWs, 33% of those exposed to COVID-19 reported depressive symptoms, 42% reported anxiety symptoms, 40% reported acute stress, 42% reported insomnia, and 37% reported burnout [33]. At our hospital, the prevalence of psychiatric symptoms among HCWs was also specifically analyzed during the pandemic through self-report surveys conducted during both waves [8]. Insomnia and anxiety were common (71.8% and 57.1%, respectively), although the frequency of both decreased in the second survey.

4.2. Underdiagnoses

The mean score on the ISI scale of the population analyzed in the present study corresponded to subclinical insomnia. Despite moderate and severe clinical insomnia being present in more than 25% of the participants, in only 3.1% of the total population was the trait of a sleep disorder detected. This frequency seems low considering the negative impact of insomnia on productivity and cognitive functioning in the medical profession [4,34,35]. Self-perceived sleep disturbances should be the first step before seeking medical evaluation, and barriers among HCWs for not doing so should be analyzed. Ideally, workplace-based interventions promoting mental health should incorporate a multidisciplinary approach to insomnia to detect it in early phases.

4.3. Interaction Between Work and Sleep

Of the 31.6% of the participants who worked overtime, less than 22% considered that these extra hours were properly paid. Low professional recognition may be linked to burnout and related symptoms [36]. A study carried out on 240 family doctors based at 70 health centers in Madrid revealed higher rates of insomnia and poorer sleep quality in those with a higher degree of burnout (39.7% vs. 7.3%) [37]. This problem needs urgent attention, as the daytime consequences of insomnia can also influence decision-making and patient care. Lack of sleep decreases the ability to discern and reflect emotions, which can reduce the clinician's ability to show empathy and engagement [34,38,39]. In addition, the incidence of errors tends to be higher among HCWs with poor mental health [40,41].

Regarding the pharmacological strategies against insomnia, 23.3% of the participants reported taking medications at least once a month to help them sleep, and more than a quarter did so without a medical prescription. These percentages appear to be higher than previously reported by Andrés-Olivera et al. [8] during the first two waves of the pandemic at our hospital. Most individuals did not take benzodiazepines (68.9%; n = 42), and no significant increase in substance use was found compared to pre-pandemic levels. According to these data, substance use by HCWs may have been aggravated after the COVID-19 pandemic. It should be noted that many of the conventional drugs used to treat insomnia (benzodiazepines, non-benzodiazepine receptor agonists, melatonin receptor agonists, and tricyclic antidepressants) present the potential for abuse and relevant adverse effects [42,43]. In contrast, new therapeutic options, such as the dual orexin receptor antagonists, have been shown to reduce excessive wakefulness and exert effects on daytime functioning [5,43,44]. Therefore, it is important to tailor the treatment of insomnia based on the socio-occupational circumstances of each individual to prevent any negative impact on both personal and professional aspects [45].

According to our findings, working shifts can be an aggravating factor for insomnia, as previously described [6,46,47]. Overtime and demanding work conditions with lengthy shifts have been described as stressful circumstances that affect resilience and mental health outcomes among HCWs [47], as well as physicians' cognitive skills and performance [48]. Flexible scheduling could enhance the sleep of physicians who work night shifts, thereby reducing their levels of fatigue and improving patient care.

Our study is subject to a series of limitations. First, the single-center design may prevent the extrapolation of our findings to other centers. Moreover, studies based on surveys may be affected by selection bias owing to the different motivations of the participants for expressing their opinions. Due to the cross-sectional design, causal effects of shift work and COVID-19 sequelae on insomnia cannot be asserted. Pre-existing mental health conditions and workload variability may have acted as confounding variables. Additional limitations may have been the potential recall bias in self-reported sleep assessments, the lack of objective sleep measures (e.g., polysomnography, actigraphy), and the lack of longitudinal data to assess causality. However, these results, which are from a large sample representing a relevant part of our center's HCWs, contribute to a field where real-world data in the work setting are scarce. They could serve as a basis for future research on the effect of strategies to manage insomnia on the work performance and daily functioning of HCWs.

5. Conclusions

Insomnia is common among HCWs and affects mental health and work performance. It could be hypothesized that the sequelae of COVID-19 and shift work could trigger or aggravate sleep disorders, exerting bidirectional effects with coexisting medical and mental disorders.

Workplace-based interventions at the organizational level promoting mental health and well-being among HCWs should incorporate a perspective on sleep problems and their consequences. Successful management requires a multidisciplinary approach, whereby specialists in neurology, psychiatry, psychology, and occupational health, among others, work on the design of joint protocols that address insomnia. Large-scale studies are needed to test multidisciplinary strategies in this setting. The physical and mental well-being of these professionals is important not only at the personal level but also to ensure that patients receive high-quality clinical care.

Supplementary Materials: The following supporting information can be downloaded at: https://www.mdpi/article/10.3390/jcm14051663/s1, Appendix S1: Sleep Screening Assessment Questionnaire; Supplementary S1: Sample size and the minimun number of participants; Supplementary S2: poster that was put on the hospital walls.

Author Contributions: C.R., J.B.-G. and A.G.-S.: planning and conducting the study, collecting data, and drafting the manuscript. All authors: interpreting study data. C.R. and A.G.-S. are equal contributors to this work and are designated as first co-authors. All authors have read and agreed to the published version of the manuscript.

Funding: The authors disclose the following financial support for the research, authorship, and/or publication of this article: an unrestricted grant from Idorsia (COCOB22A-022); funding from the Fundación Española de Patología Dual; a grant from the Plan Nacional Sobre Drogas 2022/050; a grant from the Instituto de Salud Carlos III (ISCIII) for the project' Network of Research in Primary Care of Addictions' (RD21/0009/0029), co-funded by the European Union—NextGenerationEU, Recovery and Resilience Facility (RRF). Medical writing support was provide by Medical Practice Group.

Institutional Review Board Statement: This study was conducted in accordance with the Declaration of Helsinki and approved by the Ethics Committee of IBSAL (protocol code PI 2002101152 and date of approval 10-November-2022).

Informed Consent Statement: Informed consent was obtained from all subjects involved in the study.

Data Availability Statement: The data presented in this study are available upon request from the corresponding author. The data are not publicly available due to privacy or ethical restrictions.

Conflicts of Interest: Carlos Roncero has received fees for lectures from Janssen-Cilag, Exceltis, AbbVie, Takeda, Casen-Recordati, Carnot, Angelini, Camurus, Esteve, Tecno Quimica, Viatris, and Adamed. He has received financial compensation for his participation as a consultant or a board member from Gilead, Exceltis, Camurus, AbbVie, Idorsia, Rovi, and Recordati. He carried out the PROTEUS project, which was funded by a grant from Indivior, and the COSTEDOPIA project, which was funded by Indivior. He received two medical education grants from Gilead and medical writing support from AbbVie. José Bravo has received fees for lectures from Idorsia and GSK. Pilar Andrés-Olivera has received fees for lectures from Janssen, Lundbeck, and Laboratorios Alter. Lourdes Aguilar has received fees for lectures from Casen Recordati and Viatris. Diego Remón-Gallo, Candela Payo, Alicia Fernández-Parra, Marta Peña-Ramos, and Armando González-Sánchez declare no conflicts of interest. The funders had no role in the design of the study; in the collection, analysis, or interpretation of data; in the writing of the manuscript; or in the decision to publish the results.

References

1. National Heart L and BI (NHLBI). What Are Sleep Deprivation and Deficiency? 2017. Available online: https://www.nhlbi.nih.gov/health/sleep-deprivation (accessed on 15 November 2024).
2. Stewart, N.H.; Arora, V.M. The Impact of Sleep and Circadian Disorders on Physician Burnout. *Chest* **2019**, *156*, 1022–1030. [CrossRef] [PubMed]
3. Sawadogo, W.; Adera, T.; Alattar, M.; Perera, R.; Burch, J.B. Association Between Insomnia Symptoms and Trajectory With the Risk of Stroke in the Health and Retirement Study. *Neurology* **2023**, *101*, e475–e488. [CrossRef] [PubMed]
4. Riemann, D.; Benz, F.; Dressle, R.J.; Espie, C.A.; Johann, A.F.; Blanken, T.F.; Leerssen, J.; Wassing, R.; Henry, A.L.; Kyle, S.D.; et al. Insomnia disorder: State of the science and challenges for the future. *J. Sleep Res.* **2022**, *31*, e13604. [CrossRef]
5. Jiang, F.; Li, H.; Chen, Y.; Lu, H.; Ni, J.; Chen, G. Daridorexant for the treatment of insomnia disorder: A systematic review and meta-analysis of randomized controlled trials. *Medicine* **2023**, *102*, e32754. [CrossRef]
6. Kecklund, G.; Axelsson, J. Health consequences of shift work and insufficient sleep. *BMJ* **2016**, *355*, i5210. [CrossRef] [PubMed]
7. Pappa, S.; Ntella, V.; Giannakas, T.; Giannakoulis, V.G.; Papoutsi, E.; Katsaounou, P. Prevalence of depression, anxiety, and insomnia among healthcare workers during the COVID-19 pandemic: A systematic review and meta-analysis. *Brain Behav. Immun.* **2020**, *88*, 901–907. [CrossRef]
8. Andrés-Olivera, P.; García-Aparicio, J.; López, M.T.L.; Sánchez, J.A.B.; Martín, C.; Maciá-Casas, A.; González-Sánchez, A.; Marcos, M.; Roncero, C. Impact on Sleep Quality, Mood, Anxiety, and Personal Satisfaction of Doctors Assigned to COVID-19 Units. *Int. J. Environ. Res. Public Health* **2022**, *19*, 2712. [CrossRef]
9. Roncero, C.; Díaz-Trejo, S.; Álvarez-Lamas, E.; García-Ullán, L.; Bersabé-Pérez, M.; Benito-Sánchez, J.A.; González-Sánchez, A. Follow-up of telemedicine mental health interventions amid COVID-19 pandemic. *Sci. Rep.* **2024**, *14*, 14921. [CrossRef]

10. Mortier, P.; Vilagut, G.; García-Mieres, H.; Alayo, I.; Ferrer, M.; Amigo, F.; Aragonès, E.; Aragón-Peña, A.; del Barco, Á.A.; Campos, M.; et al. Health service and psychotropic medication use for mental health conditions among healthcare workers active during the Spain COVID-19 Pandemic–A prospective cohort study using web-based surveys. *Psychiatry Res.* **2024**, *334*, 115800. [CrossRef]
11. Wang, W.; Ji, X.; Guo, H.-Y.; Tao, M.; Jin, L.; Chen, M.; Yuan, H.; Peng, H. Investigation on sleep-related cognition of Chinese health care workers during the first wave of COVID-19 pandemic. *Front. Psychiatry* **2023**, *14*, 1019837. [CrossRef]
12. Sanchez-Plazas, L.C.; García-De Jesus, R.; Martinez-Gonzalez, K.G.; Amaya-Ardila, C.P.; Almodóvar-Rivera, I.A. The psychological impact of the COVID-19 pandemic on physicians in Puerto Rico: A cross-sectional study after the second wave in 2021. *Front. Psychiatry* **2024**, *14*, 1329427. [CrossRef]
13. Gu, K.; Chen, H.; Shi, H.; Hua, C. Global prevalence of excessive daytime sleepiness among nurses: A systematic review and meta-analysis. *Int. Nurs. Rev.* **2025**, *72*, e13087. [CrossRef] [PubMed]
14. Shafiee, A.; Athar, M.M.T.; Seighali, N.; Amini, M.J.; Hajishah, H.; Bahri, R.A.; Akhoundi, A.; Beiky, M.; Sarvipour, N.; Maleki, S.; et al. The prevalence of depression, anxiety, and sleep disturbances among medical students and resident physicians in Iran: A systematic review and meta-analysis. *PLoS ONE* **2024**, *19*, e0307117. [CrossRef]
15. Zheng, J.; Jiang, M.; Zheng, K.; Li, J.; Ye, L.; Wu, J.; Feng, J.; Luo, X.; Liao, Y.; Chen, Z. Psychological Status and its Influencing Factors of Staff in a District of Shenzhen: A Retrospective Study. *Actas Esp. Psiquiatr.* **2025**, *53*, 119–125. [CrossRef] [PubMed]
16. Serrano-Ripoll, M.J.; Zamanillo-Campos, R.; Castro, A.; Fiol-de Roque, M.A.; Ricci-Cabello, I. Insomnia and sleep quality in healthcare workers fighting against COVID-19: A systematic review of the literature and meta-analysis. *Actas Esp. Psiquiatr.* **2021**, *49*, 155–179.
17. Bastien, C. Validation of the Insomnia Severity Index as an outcome measure for insomnia research. *Sleep Med.* **2001**, *2*, 297–307. [CrossRef] [PubMed]
18. Fernandez-Mendoza, J.; Rodriguez-Muñoz, A.; Vela-Bueno, A.; Olavarrieta-Bernardino, S.; Calhoun, S.L.; Bixler, E.O.; Vgontzas, A.N. The Spanish version of the Insomnia Severity Index: A confirmatory factor analysis. *Sleep Med.* **2012**, *13*, 207–210. [CrossRef]
19. Sierra, J.C.; Guillén-Serrano, V.; Santos-Iglesias, P. Insomnia Severity Index: Some indicators about its reliability and validity on an older adults sample. *Rev. Neurol.* **2008**, *47*, 566–570. [CrossRef]
20. Mills, S.D.; Fox, R.S.; Pan, T.M.; Malcarne, V.L.; Roesch, S.C.; Sadler, G.R. Psychometric Evaluation of the Patient Health Questionnaire-4 in Hispanic Americans. *Hisp. J. Behav. Sci.* **2015**, *37*, 560–571. [CrossRef]
21. Kroenke, K.; Spitzer, R.L.; Williams, J.B.W.; Lowe, B. An Ultra-Brief Screening Scale for Anxiety and Depression: The PHQ-4. *Psychosomatics* **2009**, *50*, 613–621. [CrossRef]
22. Caneo, C.; Toro, P.; Ferreccio, C. Validity and Performance of the Patient Health Questionnaire (PHQ-2) for Screening of Depression in a Rural Chilean Cohort. *Community Ment. Health J.* **2020**, *56*, 1284–1291. [CrossRef]
23. Chagas, M.H.; Crippa, J.A.; Loureiro, S.R.; Hallak, J.E.; de Meneses-Gaya, C.; Machado-De-Sousa, J.P.; Rodrigues, G.R.; Filho, A.S.; Sanches, R.F.; Tumas, V. Validity of the PHQ-2 for the screening of major depression in Parkinson's disease: Two questions and one important answer. *Aging Ment. Health* **2011**, *15*, 838–843. [CrossRef]
24. González-Sánchez, A.; Ortega-Moreno, R.; Villegas-Barahona, G.; Carazo-Vargas, E.; Arias-LeClaire, H.; Vicente-Galindo, P. New cut-off points of PHQ-9 and its variants, in Costa Rica: A nationwide observational study. *Sci. Rep.* **2023**, *13*, 14295. [CrossRef] [PubMed]
25. García-Campayo, J.; Zamorano, E.; Ruiz, M.A.; Pérez-Páramo, M.; López-Gómez, V.; Rejas, J. The assessment of generalized anxiety disorder: Psychometric validation of the Spanish version of the self-administered GAD-2 scale in daily medical practice. *Health Qual. Life Outcomes* **2012**, *10*, 114. [CrossRef]
26. Kroenke, K.; Spitzer, R.L.; Williams, J.B.W.; Monahan, P.O.; Löwe, B. Anxiety Disorders in Primary Care: Prevalence, Impairment, Comorbidity, and Detection. *Ann. Intern. Med.* **2007**, *146*, 317. [CrossRef]
27. Mitchell, A.J.; Yadegarfar, M.; Gill, J.; Stubbs, B. Case finding and screening clinical utility of the Patient Health Questionnaire (PHQ-9 and PHQ-2) for depression in primary care: A diagnostic meta-analysis of 40 studies. *BJPsych Open* **2016**, *2*, 127–138. [CrossRef]
28. IBM Corp. *IBM SPSS Statistics for Windows*, Version 28.0; IBM Corp: Armonk, NY, USA, 2021.
29. Al Maqbali, M.; Al Sinani, M.; Al-Lenjawi, B. Prevalence of stress, depression, anxiety and sleep disturbance among nurses during the COVID-19 pandemic: A systematic review and meta-analysis. *J. Psychosom. Res.* **2021**, *141*, 110343. [CrossRef]
30. Luceño-Moreno, L.; Talavera-Velasco, B.; García-Albuerne, Y.; Martín-García, J. Symptoms of Posttraumatic Stress, Anxiety, Depression, Levels of Resilience and Burnout in Spanish Health Personnel during the COVID-19 Pandemic. *Int. J. Environ. Res. Public Health* **2020**, *17*, 5514. [CrossRef]
31. Hertenstein, E.; Feige, B.; Gmeiner, T.; Kienzler, C.; Spiegelhalder, K.; Johann, A.; Jansson-Fröjmark, M.; Palagini, L.; Rücker, G.; Riemann, D.; et al. Insomnia as a predictor of mental disorders: A systematic review and meta-analysis. *Sleep Med. Rev.* **2019**, *43*, 96–105. [CrossRef] [PubMed]

32. Zhang, S.X.; Chen, R.Z.; Xu, W.; Yin, A.; Dong, R.K.; Chen, B.Z.; Delios, A.Y.; Miller, S.; McIntyre, R.S.; Ye, W.; et al. A Systematic Review and Meta-Analysis of Symptoms of Anxiety, Depression, and Insomnia in Spain in the COVID-19 Crisis. *Int. J. Environ. Res. Public Health* **2022**, *19*, 1018. [CrossRef] [PubMed]
33. Aymerich, C.; Pedruzo, B.; Pérez, J.L.; Laborda, M.; Herrero, J.; Blanco, J.; Mancebo, G.; Andrés, L.; Estévez, O.; Fernandez, M.; et al. COVID-19 pandemic effects on health worker's mental health: Systematic review and meta-analysis. *Eur. Psychiatry* **2022**, *65*, e10. [CrossRef]
34. Trockel, M.T.; Menon, N.K.; Rowe, S.G.; Stewart, M.T.; Smith, R.; Lu, M.; Kim, P.K.; Quinn, M.A.; Lawrence, E.; Marchalik, D.; et al. Assessment of Physician Sleep and Wellness, Burnout, and Clinically Significant Medical Errors. *JAMA Netw. Open* **2020**, *3*, e2028111. [CrossRef]
35. Cunningham, J.E.A.; Jones, S.A.H.; Eskes, G.A.; Rusak, B. Acute Sleep Restriction Has Differential Effects on Components of Attention. *Front. Psychiatry* **2018**, *9*, 499. [CrossRef]
36. Shanafelt, T.D.; Boone, S.; Tan, L.; Dyrbye, L.N.; Sotile, W.; Satele, D.; West, C.P.; Sloan, J.; Oreskovich, M.R. Burnout and Satisfaction With Work-Life Balance Among US Physicians Relative to the General US Population. *Arch. Intern. Med.* **2012**, *172*, 1377. [CrossRef]
37. Vela-Bueno, A.; Moreno-Jiménez, B.; Rodríguez-Muñoz, A.; Olavarrieta-Bernardino, S.; Fernández-Mendoza, J.; De la Cruz-Troca, J.J.; Bixler, E.O.; Vgontzas, A.N. Insomnia and sleep quality among primary care physicians with low and high burnout levels. *J. Psychosom. Res.* **2008**, *64*, 435–442. [CrossRef] [PubMed]
38. van der Helm, E.; Gujar, N.; Walker, M.P. Sleep Deprivation Impairs the Accurate Recognition of Human Emotions. *Sleep* **2010**, *33*, 335–342. [CrossRef]
39. Krause, A.J.; Ben Simon, E.; Mander, B.A.; Greer, S.M.; Saletin, J.M.; Goldstein-Piekarski, A.N.; Walker, M.P. The sleep-deprived human brain. *Nat. Rev. Neurosci.* **2017**, *18*, 404–418. [CrossRef]
40. Melnyk, B.M.; Tan, A.; Hsieh, A.P.; Gawlik, K.; Arslanian-Engoren, C.; Braun, L.T.; Dunbar, S.; Dunbar-Jacob, J.; Lewis, L.M.; Millan, A.; et al. Critical Care Nurses' Physical and Mental Health, Worksite Wellness Support, and Medical Errors. *Am. J. Crit. Care* **2021**, *30*, 176–184. [CrossRef]
41. Mountain, S.A.; Quon, B.S.; Dodek, P.; Sharpe, R.; Ayas, N.T. The Impact of Housestaff Fatigue on Occupational and Patient Safety. *Lung* **2007**, *185*, 203–209. [CrossRef] [PubMed]
42. Sutton, E.L. Insomnia. *Ann. Intern. Med.* **2021**, *174*, ITC33–ITC48. [CrossRef] [PubMed]
43. Shaha, D. Insomnia Management: A Review and Update. *J. Fam. Pr.* **2023**, *72*, S31. [CrossRef]
44. Rosenberg, R.; Murphy, P.; Zammit, G.; Mayleben, D.; Kumar, D.; Dhadda, S.; Filippov, G.; LoPresti, A.; Moline, M. Comparison of Lemborexant With Placebo and Zolpidem Tartrate Extended Release for the Treatment of Older Adults With Insomnia Disorder. *JAMA Netw. Open* **2019**, *2*, e1918254. [CrossRef]
45. Pérez-Carbonell, L.; Mignot, E.; Leschziner, G.; Dauvilliers, Y. Understanding and approaching excessive daytime sleepiness. *Lancet* **2022**, *400*, 1033–1046. [CrossRef]
46. Besedovsky, L.; Lange, T.; Haack, M. The Sleep-Immune Crosstalk in Health and Disease. *Physiol. Rev.* **2019**, *99*, 1325–1380. [CrossRef]
47. Manchia, M.; Gathier, A.W.; Yapici-Eser, H.; Schmidt, M.V.; de Quervain, D.; van Amelsvoort, T.; Bisson, J.I.; Cryan, J.F.; Howes, O.D.; Pinto, L.; et al. The impact of the prolonged COVID-19 pandemic on stress resilience and mental health: A critical review across waves. *Eur. Neuropsychopharmacol.* **2022**, *55*, 22–83. [CrossRef]
48. Leso, V.; Fontana, L.; Caturano, A.; Vetrani, I.; Fedele, M.; Iavicoli, I. Impact of Shift Work and Long Working Hours on Worker Cognitive Functions: Current Evidence and Future Research Needs. *Int. J. Environ. Res. Public Health* **2021**, *18*, 6540. [CrossRef]

Disclaimer/Publisher's Note: The statements, opinions and data contained in all publications are solely those of the individual author(s) and contributor(s) and not of MDPI and/or the editor(s). MDPI and/or the editor(s) disclaim responsibility for any injury to people or property resulting from any ideas, methods, instructions or products referred to in the content.

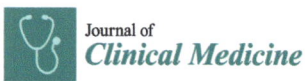

Article

Prevalence and Risk Factors of Mobile Screen Dependence in Arab Women Screened with Psychological Stress: A Cross-Talk with Demographics and Insomnia

Omar Gammoh [1,2,*], Abdelrahim Alqudah [3], Mariam Al-Ameri [2], Bilal Sayaheen [4,5], Mervat Alsous [2], Deniz Al-Tawalbeh [6], Mo'en Alnasraween [7], Batoul Al. Muhaissen [8], Alaa A. A. Aljabali [9], Sireen Abdul Rahim Shilbayeh [10] and Esam Qnais [11]

[1] Entrepreneurship and Innovation Center, Yarmouk University, Irbid 21163, Jordan
[2] Department of Clinical Pharmacy and Pharmacy Practice, Faculty of Pharmacy, Yarmouk University, Irbid 21163, Jordan; m.alameri@yu.edu.jo (M.A.-A.); mervat.alsous@yu.edu.jo (M.A.)
[3] Department of Clinical Pharmacy and Pharmacy Practice, Faculty of Pharmaceutical Sciences, The Hashemite University, Zarqa 13133, Jordan; abdelrahim@hu.edu.jo
[4] E-Learning and Open Education Resources Center, Yarmouk University, Irbid 21163, Jordan; bsayaheen@yu.edu.jo
[5] Department of Translation, Yarmouk University, Irbid 21163, Jordan
[6] Department of Medicinal Chemistry and Pharmacognosy, Faculty of Pharmacy, Yarmouk University, Irbid 21163, Jordan; deniz.altawalbeh@yu.edu.jo
[7] Department of Counseling and Educational Psychology, Faculty of Educational Sciences, Yarmouk University, Irbid 21163, Jordan; moen.na@yu.edu.jo
[8] Department of Modern Languages, Faculty of Arts, Yarmouk University, Irbid 21163, Jordan; batoul@yu.edu.jo
[9] Department of Pharmaceutics and Pharmaceutical Technology, Faculty of Pharmacy, Yarmouk University, Irbid 21163, Jordan; alaaj@yu.edu.jo
[10] Department of Pharmacy Practice, College of Pharmacy, Princess Nourah bint Abdulrahman University, P.O. Box 84428, Riyadh 11671, Saudi Arabia; ssabdulrahim@pnu.edu.sa
[11] Department of Biology and Biotechnology, Faculty of Science, The Hashemite University, Zarqa 13133, Jordan; esamqn@hu.edu.jo
* Correspondence: omar.gammoh@yu.edu.jo

Abstract: Background/Objectives: The current study aims to investigate the rate and the factors associated with mobile screen dependence as a coping mechanism among women residing in Jordan and screened for stress, with a focus on demographics and insomnia. **Methods**: This cross-sectional study with predefined inclusion criteria used validated tools to assess stress, anxiety, and insomnia. **Results**: The data analyzed from 431 women showed that 265 (61.5%) were ≤25 years old, 352 (81.7%) received a university education, and 201 (46.6%) were current students. In addition, 207 (48.0%) reported a dependence on mobile screens for coping, 107 (24.8%) reported severe anxiety, and 180 (41.7%) reported severe insomnia. The multivariable regression analysis revealed that mobile screen dependence—as a personal coping choice—was significantly associated with "students" (OR = 1.75, 95% CI = 1.19–2.57, $p = 0.004$) and "severe insomnia" (OR = 1.07, 95% CI = 1.07–2.32, $p = 0.02$). **Conclusions**: We report that a high rate of mobile dependence is associated with students and insomnia. Prompt action should be taken to raise awareness regarding the proper coping mechanisms in this population.

Keywords: Jordan; women; mental health; mobile screens

1. Introduction

Screen addiction is a cognitive behavior addiction characterized by excessive phone use and dependence. According to the official website of the Department of Statistics in Jordan, the population of the Hashemite kingdom was estimated to be 11,516,000 at the end of 2023, with females comprising 47.1% of the total. Additionally, Jordan is a youthful country, with one-fifth of its population falling within the youth category, specifically in the age group of 15–24 years, according to a recent report on population estimates prepared by the Department of Statistics in Jordan. In this context, the UNICEF Jordan official website indicates that 63% of Jordan's population is under the age of 30 [1].

In this technologized era, youths depend on screens—whether smartphones, tablets, or televisions—daily for various purposes, including entertainment, study, and work. The improper excessive use of screens can result in various physical, mental, and psychological/behavioral concerns, including sleep disorders, eye problems, neck and back problems, anxiety, and depression, among many others [2–4].

Screens can also serve as a coping mechanism to avoid or manage stressful situations, particularly given the vast amount of news distributed through various social media platforms. Although Jordan has been a safe zone amid armed conflicts for more than a decade, news reports continue to contribute to stress, anxiety, and insomnia among people in the region, including those in Jordan [4,5].

Insomnia is a common sleep disorder characterized by poor sleep quality, latency sleep, and frequent awakening. Insomnia is tightly related to stress, anxiety, and other mental health disorders. Women are more likely to report insomnia [6]. Insomnia and mobile screen dependence are closely related. Evidence from cross-sectional studies in Jordan suggests a bi-directional relationship between them [7].

Women are more vulnerable to experiencing mental health disturbances due to many physiological and environmental stressors, especially in developing countries. This includes hormonal changes, the duties of daily life, and responsibilities including work, study, household work, and others [8]. For example, evidence shows that insomnia and its related problems are higher in women compared to men [6].

Long-term psychological stress is tightly related to mental and behavioral impairments that affect the daily functioning of individuals, especially women [9]. For instance, stress is associated with several somatic immune-related diseases, depression, anxiety, and insomnia [10,11].

Although several investigations have been published about smartphone overuse and mobile screen dependence, to our knowledge, no previous studies have been completely dedicated to investigating this behavior among women screened for stress in Jordan.

The current study aimed to investigate the rate and factors associated with mobile screen dependence as a coping mechanism among women screened for stress in Jordan, with a focus on demographics and insomnia.

2. Materials and Methods

2.1. Study Design and Settings

The present study followed a cross-sectional design and recruited a sample of Jordanian women according to predefined inclusion criteria through social media platforms related to Yarmouk University. The researchers uploaded the study tool on a Google Form and applied the snowball sampling technique. The objective and steps of the study were all explained to the potential participants before they chose to enroll and approved the consent form. The study obtained approval from Yarmouk University's IRB committee (number 479). All participants signed an online consent form before enrolling in the study.

2.2. Inclusion Criteria

Females aged 18 years old, residing in Jordan, willing to participate, and screened for significant stress using the Perceived Stress Scale (PSS) were included. In brief, the Arabic version of the Perceived Stress Scale, originally developed by Cohen [12], was used. It comprises 14 items designed to measure individual stress over the past month, with a cut-off score of ≥ 15 reflecting clinically significant stress, as supported by previous research [13].

2.3. Exclusion Criteria

Women with a stress score of less than 15 and presenting incomplete or missing data were excluded.

2.4. Study Instrument

The study instrument consisted of three distinct sections: demographics, insomnia, and anxiety. The demographics section included structured questions about the participants' age, marital status, education, employment, and smoking status. This section also included the outcome variable 'mobile dependence', through a question identifying stress coping options. The question was formulated as follows: 'To relieve stress, I depend on "my mobile" or other choices such as sports, eating, and others'. Participants were free to select one or more options.

2.5. Anxiety

The severity of anxiety in the sample was assessed using the validated and reliable Arabic version of the General Anxiety Disorder-7 (GAD-7). This self-administered scale consists of 7 questions that assess symptoms of anxiety over the past fourteen days. The scale has a sensitivity of 89% and a specificity of 82% for diagnosing generalized anxiety disorder. For example, questions include 'Feeling nervous, anxious, or on edge?', 'Worrying too much about different things?', 'Feeling afraid, as if something awful might happen?', with response options 'not at all = 0' to 'nearly every day = 3'. Respondents with a score of ≥ 15 were classified as having severe anxiety symptoms [14,15].

2.6. Insomnia

The severity of insomnia was assessed using the translated, validated, and reliable (Cronbach alpha = 0.81) Insomnia Severity Index–Arabic (ISI-A). The ISI-A assesses insomnia severity and its impact on daily life activities over the past 14 days. It consists of seven questions and generates a maximum score of 28. For example, questions include the following: 'difficulty falling asleep?', 'difficulty staying asleep?', and 'problems walking up too early?', with answers ranging from 'none = 0', to 'very = 4". Participants scoring 15 or above are considered to have severe insomnia [16,17].

2.7. Data Analysis

The data presented were categorical and were therefore summarized as frequencies and percentages, as shown in Table 1. To identify which independent variables were associated with mobile screen dependence (dependent variable), a preparatory univariate analysis was conducted (Table 2), followed by a multivariable binary regression analysis, where only significant variables ($p < 0.05$) were retained in the final model. Data were analyzed using SPSS software version 21. The confidence interval was set at 95%, and the significance level was set at $p < 0.05$.

Table 1. Study sample characteristics (n = 431).

Factor	Category	N (%)
Age (Years)	≤25	265 (61.5)
	>25	166 (38.5)
Marital status	Single	267 (61.9)
	Married	147 (34.1)
	Divorced	13 (3.0)
	Widow	4 (0.9)
Education level	Primary school	2 (0.5)
	Secondary school	33 (7.7)
	University	352 (81.7)
	Postgraduate study	44 (10.2)
Employment status	Does not work	111 (25.8)
	Student	201 (46.6)
	Work	105 (24.4)
	Retired	14 (3.2)
Smoking status	Non-smoker	352 (81.7)
	Smoker	79 (18.3)
	Use E-cigarette	22 (5.1)
	Use Shisha	56 (13.0)
	Negative smoker	51 (11.8)
Having chronic diseases	Yes	54 (12.5)
	No	377 (87.5)
Screen dependent	Yes	207 (48.0)
	No	224 (52.0)
Severe Insomnia		180 (41.7)
Severe Anxiety		107 (24.8)

Table 2. Univariate analysis of risk factors associated with mobile screen dependence (N = 431).

	Use Screen (N = 207) N (%)	Do Not Use Screens (N = 224) N (%)	p-Value
Age			
≤25	142 (68.6)	123 (54.9)	0.004 *
>25	65 (31.4)	101 (45.1)	
Marital status			
Single	140 (67.6)	127 (56.7)	
Married	61 (29.5)	86 (38.4)	0.040 *
Widow	0 (0.0)	4 (1.8)	
Divorced	6 (2.9)	7 (3.1)	

Table 2. *Cont.*

	Use Screen (N = 207) N (%)	Do Not Use Screens (N = 224) N (%)	*p*-Value
Employment status			
Work	42 (20.3)	69 (30.8)	
Does not work	50 (24.2)	55 (24.6)	0.004 *
Student	112 (54.1)	89 (39.7)	
Retired	3 (1.4)	11 (4.9)	
Educational level			
Primary	1 (0.4)	2 (0.4)	
Secondary	12 (5.5)	21 (9.4)	0.356
University level	176 (85.0)	176 (78.6)	
Postgraduate study	18 (8.7)	26 (11.6)	
Living Place			
Inside Amman	26 (12.6)	30 (13.4)	0.797
Outside Amman	181 (87.4)	194 (86.6)	
Smoking			
Not smoker	166 (80.2)	186 (83.0)	0.446
Smoker	41 (19.8)	38 (17.0)	
Having chronic diseases			
Yes	30 (14.5)	24 (10.7)	0.236
No	177 (85.5)	200 (89.3)	
Having severe insomnia			
Yes	99 (47.8)	81 (36.2)	0.014 *
No	108 (52.2)	143 (63.8)	
Having anxiety			
Yes	57 (27.5)	50 (22.3)	0.211
No	150 (72.5)	174 (77.7)	

* *p*-value < 0.05.

3. Results

3.1. Study Sample Characteristics

The total number of responders was 612. After applying the inclusion criteria, the number was reduced to 431. The results showed that 265 (61.5%) were ≤25 years old, 267 (61.9%) were single, 352 (81.7%) received a university education, 201 (46.6%) were students, 352 (81.7%) identified themselves as non-smokers, and 377 (87.5) reported no long-term health conditions. In addition, 207 (48.0%) reported depending on mobile screens for coping, while 107 (24.8%) reported severe anxiety and 180 (41.7%) reported severe insomnia (Table 1).

3.2. Risk Factors Associated with Mobile Screen Dependence

The preparatory univariate regression analysis (Table 2) revealed the following independent variables as potential confounders: 'age', 'marital status', 'employment', and 'insomnia'.

These variables were used to create the multivariable binary regression model, as shown in Table 3, which revealed that the dependent variable 'mobile screens dependence' was significantly associated with 'students' (OR = 1.75, 95% CI = 1.19–2.57, p = 0.004) and 'severe insomnia' (OR = 1.07, 95% CI = 1.07–2.32, p = 0.02).

Table 3. Binary logistic regression analysis of risk factors associated with mobile screen dependence.

Independent Variable	B	SE	Odds Ratio	95% CI	p-Value
Being a student	0.558	0.197	1.748	1.19–2.57	0.004 *
Having severe insomnia	0.453	0.199	1.572	1.07–2.32	0.023 *

* p-value < 0.05. B, regression coefficient; SE, standard error associated with the coefficient B; CI, confidence interval.

4. Discussion

The current study aimed to investigate the rate and risk factors associated with mobile screen dependence as a coping mechanism among Jordanian women screened for stress. According to our results, almost half of the women reported choosing mobile screens as their primary coping mechanism to relieve stress and anxiety. Additionally, mobile screen dependence among women was significantly associated with being a student and experiencing severe insomnia. To our knowledge, this is the first study to highlight the risk factors associated with mobile screen dependence among women residing in Jordan. Despite the importance of women's well-being, this topic remains relatively overlooked in many settings.

The study revealed significant correlations between having a dependence on mobile devices and specific variables, such as being a student and having acute insomnia. Students were 1.75 times more likely than non-students to be dependent on mobile screens. This finding is supported by the literature; according to Liu et al., 52.8% of medical students were found to be addicted to smartphones [18]. Another study on smartphone addiction among undergraduates found that 49% of respondents used their phones for at least five hours daily [19]. A recent review explored the reasons for mobile screen addiction among students. In contemporary student life, smartphones serve as platforms for communication and entertainment, in addition to being academic tools. The younger generation extensively uses smartphones for social networking, studying, entertainment, and internet browsing [20].

The use of smartphones as an essential tool is increasing in people's daily lives. These devices allow people to access information, interact with friends, and manage daily tasks with ease and convenience. Smartphones offer numerous advantages as multi-purpose tools for communication, education, entertainment, and achieving business goals. Despite these advantages and the strong reliance on these devices, increased daily use poses several potential future risks [21].

Some of these risks may affect long-term cognitive functioning, which may hinder students' ability to maintain focus and engage in deep learning processes. According to a study by Ophir et al. (2009) [22], habitual multitasking—often driven by smartphone technology—can lead to a loss of cognitive control and reduce task management effectiveness. In an increasingly complex and demanding world, these consequences may make hinder children's academic and professional success [23].

The decline in interpersonal communication skills is another potential risk. The instant communication made possible by smartphones has reduced personal encounters, weakening social ties and emotional intelligence. Furthermore, increased screen use has been linked to decreased psychological well-being, as shown by longitudinal research such as that conducted by Twenge and Campbell (2018) [21]. This raises questions about the state of students' mental health in a world where digital settings are prevalent. In this context, Livingstone and Smith (2014) pointed out that the misuse of smartphone technology—such as cyberbullying or exposure to harmful content—can have lasting psychological effects [23].

People often check their smartphones in the evening, even during long and stressful work days. However, this behavior can disrupt sleeping habits and patterns, as individuals forgets the time while scrolling through social media pages. In addition, the blue light emitted by smart devices negatively affects the brain's daily rhythm, tricking it into thinking that it is still early, which can lead to insomnia over time [24].

The continuous use of these devices may harm the eyes and weaken vision. It can also harm the neck and spine. Digital screens emit blue light, which harms eye health and vision. The deterioration of the psychological state of many individuals is accompanied by anxiety or tension as they spend more hours on smartphones, further increasing the risks resulting from this use.

The study also finds a strong correlation between mobile screen dependence and severe insomnia. The likelihood of relying on mobile screens was shown to be higher among those with severe insomnia. These findings align with several previous studies. For example, one study using data from a national health survey of college and university students in Norway found a significant negative correlation between sleep and screen use. These results suggest that students' screen time significantly impacts both the duration and quality of their sleep. The findings also show a significant correlation between social media addiction and increased rates of sleeplessness [25]. Additionally, several studies have proven that university students who rely heavily on their phones are more likely to experience a poor sleep quality [26,27]. One explanation for this relationship is that exposure to the blue light emitted by screens disturbs sleeping patterns by interfering with melatonin production and circadian rhythms [28].

Moreover, mobile screens can be used by individuals with insomnia as a coping mechanism or to pass time, which exacerbates sleep disturbance [29]. Social media and entertainment content on mobile devices can overstimulate the mind, making it difficult to relax and obtain restful sleep [30]. Thus, being a student with insomnia creates a vicious circle in which an excessive reliance on mobile screens both causes and results in sleep disturbances. To mitigate the detrimental effects of insomnia and mobile screen dependence, it is crucial to address screen time habits and promote improved sleep hygiene, particularly among students.

This work tackles a new and pressing topic regarding women's mental health and mobile screen dependence during times of armed conflict in the Middle East. The current work provides several strengths, such as the type of the sample and the geographical location (adjacent to zones of armed conflicts). In addition, the current work used a representative sample size, validated measurement tools, and robust data analysis. On the other hand, the cross-sectional design of the study limits our ability to establish causal relationships between variables. Additionally, the self-administered quantitative approach limited accurate diagnosis or qualitative investigation. Another limitation was the lack of information about the content accessed through mobile screens by the respondents. These limitations will be taken into consideration for future research, which will focus on the causes of stress in this population segment, i.e., young women residing in Jordan. This could include further in-depth qualitative studies to unravel any unseen causes of this disabling phenomenon and larger-scale quantitative studies conducted across several geographical locations. Additionally, future studies should address insomnia among women in Jordan. This could involve awareness sessions in universities that highlight the importance of high-quality sleep and the need to consult health care professionals to adequately manage this issue.

5. Conclusions

In conclusion, mobile dependency was found to be prevalent among Jordanian women, and was primarily associated with university students and insomnia. The rationale and the beneficial use of technology must be promoted in Jordan to enhance mental health and improve the overall well-being of women during times of stress. The findings of this research pave the way for further qualitative and quantitative studies dedicated to unravelling the causes of stress and related issues, such as insomnia, in this young and fragile population that relies heavily on technology.

Author Contributions: Conceptualization, O.G., D.A.-T. and A.A.; methodology, M.A.-A.; software, B.S.; validation, D.A.-T. and M.A. (Mervat Alsous); formal analysis, M.A. (Mervat Alsous) and B.A.M.; investigation, D.A.-T. and A.A.; resources, S.A.R.S.; data curation, M.A. (Mervat Alsous) and E.Q.; writing—original draft preparation, O.G., A.A., B.S., M.A.-A., M.A. (Mo'en Alnasraween) and A.A.A.A.; writing—review and editing, E.Q.; visualization, B.A.M., M.A. (Mo'en Alnasraween), B.S. and S.A.R.S.; supervision, E.Q., O.G. and M.A.-A.; project administration, D.A.-T. and A.A.A.A.; funding acquisition, S.A.R.S. and O.G. All authors have read and agreed to the published version of the manuscript.

Funding: Princess Nourah bint Abdulrahman University Researchers Supporting Project number (PNURSP2025R814).

Institutional Review Board Statement: The study obtained approval from Yarmouk University IRB committee (number 479 dated 17 October 2024).

Informed Consent Statement: Informed consent was obtained from all subjects involved in the study.

Data Availability Statement: Data will be made available upon reasonable request.

Acknowledgments: The current work was supported by Princess Nourah bint Abdulrahman University Researchers Supporting Project number (PNURSP2025R814), Princess Nourah bint Abdulrahman University, P.O. Box 84428, Riyadh 11671, Saudi Arabia.

Conflicts of Interest: The authors declare no conflicts of interest.

References

1. Department of Statistics. Population—Department of Statistics. 2024. Available online: https://dosweb.dos.gov.jo/population/population-2/ (accessed on 2 January 2025).
2. Wang, B.; Yao, N.; Zhou, X.; Liu, J.; Lv, Z. The association between attention deficit/hyperactivity disorder and internet addiction: A systematic review and meta-analysis. *BMC Psychiatry* **2017**, *17*, 260. [CrossRef]
3. Shi, X.; Wang, A.; Zhu, Y. Longitudinal associations among smartphone addiction, loneliness, and depressive symptoms in college students: Disentangling between–and within–person associations. *Addict. Behav.* **2023**, *142*, 107676. [CrossRef] [PubMed]
4. Gammoh, O.S.; Alqudah, A.; Qnais, E.; Alotaibi, B.S. Factors associated with insomnia and fatigue symptoms during the outbreak of Oct. 7th war on Gaza: A study from Jordan. *Prev. Med. Rep.* **2024**, *41*, 102685. [CrossRef] [PubMed]
5. MBlake, J.; Trinder, J.A.; Allen, N.B. *Mechanisms Underlying the Association Between Insomnia, Anxiety, and Depression in Adolescence: Implications for Behavioral Sleep Interventions*; Elsevier Ltd.: Amsterdam, The Netherlands, 2018; Volume 63. [CrossRef]
6. Zuo, L.; Chen, X.; Liu, M.; Dong, S.; Chen, L.; Li, G.; Zhai, Z.; Zhou, L.; Chen, H.; Wei, Y.; et al. Gender differences in the prevalence of and trends in sleep patterns and prescription medications for insomnia among US adults, 2005 to 2018. *Sleep Health* **2022**, *8*, 691–700. [CrossRef]
7. Al Battashi, N.; Al Omari, O.; Sawalha, M.; Al Maktoumi, S.; Alsuleitini, A.; Al Qadire, M. The Relationship Between Smartphone Use, Insomnia, Stress, and Anxiety Among University Students: A Cross-Sectional Study. *Clin. Nurs. Res.* **2021**, *30*, 734–740. [CrossRef]
8. Lee, M.F.; Lai, C.S. Mental Health Level and Happiness Index among Female Teachers in Malaysia. *Ann. Trop. Med. Public Health* **2020**, *23*, 231–304. [CrossRef]
9. Alshdaifat, E.; Absy, N.; Sindiani, A.; AlOsta, N.; Hijazi, H.; Amarin, Z.; Alnazly, E. Premenstrual Syndrome and Its Association with Perceived Stress: The Experience of Medical Students in Jordan. *Int. J. Women's Health* **2022**, *14*, 777–785. [CrossRef] [PubMed]

10. Stojanovich, L.; Marisavljevich, D. Stress as a trigger of autoimmune disease. *J. Neurol. Sci.* **2018**, *26*, 209–213. [CrossRef]
11. Kolahkaj, B.; Zargar, F. Effect of Mindfulness-Based Stress Reduction on Anxiety, Depression and Stress in Women with Multiple Sclerosis. *Nurs. Midwifery Stud.* **2015**, *4*, e29655. [CrossRef] [PubMed]
12. Cohen, S.; Kamarck, T.; Mermelstein, R. Perceived stress scale. *Meas. Stress A Guid. Health Soc. Sci.* **1994**, *10*, 1–2.
13. OGammoh, O.S.; Al-Smadi, A.; Alqudah, A.; Al-Habahbeh, S.; Weshah, F.; Ennab, W.; Al-Shudifat, A.E.; Bjørk, M.H. The association between fingolimod and mental health outcomes in a cohort of Multiple Sclerosis patients with stress. *Eur. Rev. Med. Pharmacol. Sci.* **2023**, *27*, 13.
14. Lo, B. Validation and Standardization of the Generalized Anxiety Disorder Screener (GAD-7) in the General Population. *Med. Care* **2008**, *46*, 266–274.
15. Gammoh, O.; Al-Smadi, A.; Mansour, M.; Ennab, W.; Al Hababbeh, S.; Al-Taani, G.; Alsous, M.; Aljabali, A.A.; Tambuwala, M.M. The relationship between psychiatric symptoms and the use of levetiracetam in people with epilepsy. *Int. J. Psychiatry Med.* **2023**, *59*, 360–372. [CrossRef] [PubMed]
16. KSuleiman, H.; Yates, B.C. Translating the insomnia severity index into Arabic. *J. Nurs. Scholarsh.* **2011**, *43*, 49–53. [CrossRef]
17. Morin, C. Insomnia: Psychological Assessment and Management. 1993. Available online: https://psycnet.apa.org/record/1993-98362-000 (accessed on 2 November 2019).
18. Liu, H.; Zhou, Z.; Huang, L.; Zhu, E.; Yu, L.; Zhang, M. Prevalence of smartphone addiction and its effects on subhealth and insomnia: A cross-sectional study among medical students. *BMC Psychiatry* **2022**, *22*, 305. [CrossRef] [PubMed]
19. Boumosleh, J.; Jaalouk, D. Smartphone addiction among university students and its relationship with academic performance. *Glob. J. Health Sci.* **2018**, *10*, 48–59. [CrossRef]
20. Zhou, B.; Mui, L.G.; Li, J.; Yang, Y.; Hu, J. A model for risk factors harms and of smartphone addiction among nursing students: A scoping review. *Nurse Educ. Pract.* **2024**, *75*, 103874. [CrossRef]
21. Twenge, J.M.; Campbell, W.K. Associations between screen time and lower psychological well-being among children and adolescents: Evidence from a population-based study. *Prev. Med. Rep.* **2018**, *12*, 271–283. [CrossRef] [PubMed]
22. Ophir, E.; Nass, C.; Wagner, A.D. Cognitive control in media multitaskers. *Proc. Natl. Acad. Sci. USA* **2009**, *106*, 15583–15587. [CrossRef] [PubMed]
23. Livingstone, S.; Smith, P.K. Annual research review: Harms experienced by child users of online and mobile technologies: The nature, prevalence and management of sexual and aggressive risks in the digital age. *J. Child Psychol. Psychiatry* **2014**, *55*, 635–654. [CrossRef] [PubMed]
24. Sohn, S.Y.; Rees, P.; Wildridge, B.; Kalk, N.J.; Carter, B. Prevalence of problematic smartphone usage and associated mental health outcomes amongst children and young people: A systematic review, meta-analysis and GRADE of the evidence. *BMC Psychiatry* **2019**, *19*, 356.
25. Gellis, L.A.; Lichstein, K.L.; Scarinci, I.C.; Durrence, H.H.; Taylor, D.J.; Bush, A.J.; Riedel, B.W. Socioeconomic status and insomnia. *J. Abnorm. Psychol.* **2005**, *114*, 111. [CrossRef]
26. Ghosh, T.; Sarkar, D.; Sarkar, K.; Dalai, C.K.; Ghosal, A. A study on smartphone addiction and its effects on sleep quality among nursing students in a municipality town of West Bengal. *J. Fam. Med. Prim. Care* **2021**, *10*, 378–386. [CrossRef] [PubMed]
27. Sohn, S.Y.; Krasnoff, L.; Rees, P.; Kalk, N.J.; Carter, B. The association between smartphone addiction and sleep: A UK cross-sectional study of young adults. *Front. Psychiatry* **2021**, *12*, 629407. [CrossRef]
28. Bonmati-Carrion, M.A.; Arguelles-Prieto, R.; Martinez-Madrid, M.J.; Reiter, R.; Hardeland, R.; Rol, M.A.; Madrid, J.A. Protecting the melatonin rhythm through circadian healthy light exposure. *Int. J. Mol. Sci.* **2014**, *15*, 23448–23500. [CrossRef] [PubMed]
29. SBauducco; Pillion, M.; Bartel, K.; Reynolds, C.; Kahn, M.; Gradisar, M. A bidirectional model of sleep and technology use: A theoretical review of How much, for whom, and which mechanisms. *Sleep Med. Rev.* **2024**, *76*, 101933. [CrossRef] [PubMed]
30. Bengtsson, S.; Johansson, S. The meanings of social media use in everyday life: Filling empty slots, everyday transformations, and mood management. *Soc. Media + Soc.* **2022**, *8*, 20563051221130292. [CrossRef]

Disclaimer/Publisher's Note: The statements, opinions and data contained in all publications are solely those of the individual author(s) and contributor(s) and not of MDPI and/or the editor(s). MDPI and/or the editor(s) disclaim responsibility for any injury to people or property resulting from any ideas, methods, instructions or products referred to in the content.

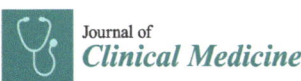

Article

Insomnia Symptoms, Mental Health Diagnosis, Mental Health Care Utilization, and Perceived Barriers in U.S. Males and Females

Wendemi Sawadogo [1,*], Anuli Njoku [1] and Joy Jegede [2]

[1] Department of Public Health, College of Health and Human Services, Southern Connecticut State University, New Haven, CT 06515, USA; njokua3@southernct.edu
[2] Department of Social Work, College of Health and Human Services, Southern Connecticut State University, New Haven, CT 06515, USA; jegedej1@southernct.edu
* Correspondence: sawadogow1@southernct.edu

Abstract: Objective: We aim to determine the association between insomnia symptoms and mental health in females and males and compare mental health care utilization and perceived barriers between females and males with insomnia symptoms. **Methods**: This is a cross-sectional study using the National Health Interview Survey. Insomnia symptoms included self-reported "trouble falling asleep", 'trouble staying asleep", and "waking up feeling not well rested". Mental health included self-reported anxiety and depression. Multivariable logistic regression was used to assess the association between insomnia symptoms and mental health in females and males. **Results**: A total of 26,691 adults were included. The mean age was 48.2 years; 51.4% were females, and 48.6% were males. Insomnia symptoms were associated with anxiety and depression for both females and males. These associations were stronger in younger adults (<50 years) than older adults (≥50 years). Females with insomnia symptoms were more likely to receive mental health care (OR = 1.7; 95% CI = 1.53, 1.87) but also to delay mental health care because of its cost (OR = 1.96; 95% CI: 1.67, 2.30) or needed mental health care but did not get it because of the cost (OR = 2.14; 95% CI: 1.82, 2.50) than their males counterpart. **Conclusions**: Insomnia symptoms were associated with mental health in females and males, being stronger in younger adults than older adults, with gender differences in mental health care utilization and financial barriers to mental health care. Holistic approaches involving prevention and better access to mental health care are warranted.

Keywords: insomnia symptoms; mental health; mental health care; anxiety; depression; females; males; health disparities

1. Introduction

The growing prevalence of mental health disorders that affect individuals' physical and social well-being makes mental health a public health issue in the United States. It is estimated that more than one in five U.S. adults live with a mental illness (59.3 million in 2022; 23.1% of the U.S. adult population) [1]. Anxiety and depression are the most common mental health disorders in the U.S. During 2022, about one in five adults age 18 and older experienced any symptoms of anxiety (18.2%) or depression (21.4%) in the past two weeks [2]. Despite the burden of mental health, access to mental health care remains a challenge, with only 47% of adults with mental illness receiving treatment [1]. Cost is the most common barrier, with over 60% of adults citing it as a reason for not seeking care.

A lack of insurance, stigma, and lack of access to health care providers are also significant barriers [3,4].

Insomnia is an experience associated with persistent difficulty initiating sleep, difficulty maintaining sleep, or waking up too early, despite adequate opportunity to sleep [5,6]. About 10% of the adult population experiences chronic insomnia, and 30% experience short-term insomnia [7]. Insomnia and sleep disorders in general constitute significant public health challenges, resulting in high health care costs while reducing work productivity.

The relationship between mental health and insomnia is complex; mental health is commonly associated with insomnia and vice versa [8]. The human body is designed to require a regular pattern for sleep, a necessary biological function to ensure healthy cognition, emotional, mental, and social well-being [5]. Insomnia disrupts this biological function and may stand as an isolated disorder, a co-occurring condition with a mental disorder, or a consequence of a mental disorder [9]. Previous longitudinal studies have reported a correlation between insomnia and depression [10,11]. A meta-analysis of longitudinal studies reported that insomnia was associated with a 3-fold increased risk of presenting anxiety disorder (pooled OR: 3.23; CI 1.52–6.85) [12]. In another meta-analysis of longitudinal studies, insomnia symptoms were independently associated with depression (pooled RR: 2.27; 95% CI: 1.89–2.71) [13]. The experience of insomnia could trigger depressive symptoms where they were previously absent.

While sex differences in insomnia patterns, on one hand, and mental health disorders, on the other hand, have been separately reported, few studies have investigated whether the association between insomnia and mental health differs by sex [14–17]. Differences between females and males were reported in the prevalence and incidence of sleep disorders and mental health. Females are more likely to report insomnia symptoms, receive a diagnosis of insomnia, and are more frequently diagnosed with mental health disorders such as anxiety and depression than males [14–17]. Suggested reasons include biological, hormonal, psychosocial, and socioeconomic factors. For example, sex hormones exert a significant influence on circadian rhythms and sleep, with estrogen, testosterone, and progesterone all playing a role in regulating sleep–wake cycles, mood, and other physiological processes [18]. It is, however, unclear if the association between insomnia symptoms and mental health differs by sex. We hypothesized that those differences would be reflected in the association between insomnia symptoms and mental health and, thus, require separate investigation. Targeted interventions may contribute to addressing the complex yet increasing mental health burden. Furthermore, males and females with insomnia symptoms may face different barriers to accessing mental health care. Using cross-sectional data representative of the U.S. adult population, this study aimed to address four objectives. First, we examined the association between insomnia symptoms and mental health in females and males. Second, we explored the moderating role of race and ethnicity, place of residence, and age. Third, we compared mental health care utilization and perceived barriers between females and males with insomnia symptoms. Fourth, we investigated potential moderation and mediation by place of residence and insurance coverage.

2. Materials and Methods

2.1. Data Source and Study Design

This cross-sectional study used publicly available and de-identified data from the 2022 National Health Interview Survey (NHIS) [19]. NHIS is an annual household survey representative of the civilian noninstitutionalized population in the United States conducted by the National Center for Health Statistics (NCHS) of the Centers for Disease Control and Prevention (CDC). To that end, the NHIS uses a complex sample design involving stratification and clustering. The main objective of the NHIS is to monitor the health of the

United States population through the collection and analysis of data on a broad range of health topics.

The survey is conducted continuously throughout the year. Interviews are conducted in respondents' homes and/or over the telephone. Informed consent is obtained from the participants. Information about the Sample Adult is self-reported, unless physically or mentally unable to do so, then a knowledgeable proxy answers for the Sample Adult. This study used data from the Sample Adults (age $\geq$ 18 years). In 2022, there were 27,651 Sample Adult interviews. The 2022 survey included, in the Sample Adult, items related to sleep and mental health assessment for depression and anxiety. As these items were rotating and not included in all surveys, the 2022 survey was appropriate for this research question.

2.2. Insomnia Symptoms

Participants were asked "during the past 30 days, how often did you wake up feeling well-rested?"; "how often did you have trouble falling asleep?"; and "how often did you have trouble staying asleep?". The response options were "never", "some days", "most days", "every day", "refused", and "don't know". Those who endorsed "never" received a score of 0, "some days" a score of 1, "most days" a score of 2, and "every day" a score of 3. Missing values were assigned to "refused" and "don't know". Reverse coding was used for the question related to "wake up feeling well-rested". The total insomnia score ranges from 0 to 9 with higher scores indicating severe insomnia symptoms.

2.3. Mental Health

Dichotomous variables were created for mental health diagnosis based on the answers to questions related to anxiety (Have you ever been told by a doctor or other health professional that you had any type of anxiety disorder?) and depression (Have you ever been told by a doctor or other health professional that you had any type of depression?). Similarly, mental health care utilization and perceived barriers were based on the following questions: "during the past 12 months, did you receive counseling or therapy from a mental health professional such as a psychiatrist, psychologist, psychiatric nurse, or clinical social worker?", "have you delayed getting counseling or therapy from a mental health professional because of the cost?", and "was there any time when you needed counseling or therapy from a mental health professional but did not get it because of the cost?".

2.4. Covariates

Based on the literature review and the available data, the covariates included age, sex (male or female), race and ethnicity (Hispanic, Non-Hispanic Asian, Non-Hispanic Black, Non-Hispanic White, and Other), education level (less than high school, high school graduate, some college, associate, bachelor, and graduate degree), marital status (married, in couple, or neither), ratio of family income to poverty threshold, smoking (current, former, or never), alcohol consumption (current, former, or abstainer), physical activity (inactive, insufficiently active, or sufficiently active), body mass index (underweight, normal weight, overweight, or obese), diabetes (yes or no), hypertension (yes or no), heart disease (yes or no), stroke (yes or no), cancer (yes or no), and sleeping pill utilization.

2.5. Statistical Analysis

Descriptive statistics were used to summarize the participants' characteristics by insomnia symptom scores. Correlations between categorical variables were assessed using the phi coefficient. Multicollinearity was tested using the variance inflation factor. Logistic regressions were developed to assess the association between insomnia symptoms and anxiety, as well as the association between insomnia symptoms and depression in males and females in the study population. In addition, logistic regression models were developed to compare mental health care utilization and perceived barriers in males and females with insomnia symptoms. This analysis was restricted to those with insomnia symptoms, as they are the ones most likely to seek health care. Moderation was assessed by adding a multiplicative interaction term in the model. Mediation was assessed using the counterfactual framework, which decomposed the total effect into natural indirect and direct effects [20]. The mediated proportion was computed as the natural indirect effect divided by the total effect, and the 95% CI was estimated by repeating 1000 bootstrapped samples. The models were adjusted for the covariates listed above. The model fit was checked using the Hosmer–Lemeshow goodness-of-fit test. Further analysis was conducted for individual insomnia symptoms by categorizing each insomnia symptom into two groups. All statistical analyses were performed in SAS® 9.4 software with an alpha level set at 0.05 (SAS Institute Inc., Cary, NC, USA).

3. Results

3.1. Description of Study Participants

A total of 26,691 adults who responded to the insomnia questions were included in the present analysis. The mean age was 48.2 years (95% CI: 47.9, 48.5), 51.4% were females and 48.6% were males (Table 1). Insomnia symptom scores were higher in females, Non-Hispanic Whites, those with a low income, smokers, those who were physically inactive, those with a high BMI, and with any comorbidity such as diabetes, hypertension, heart disease, stroke, and cancer.

Table 1. Baseline characteristics by insomnia symptom scores.

Characteristics	Insomnia Symptom Scores			
	0 n (Weighted%) [a]: 2944 (11.1)	1–4 n (Weighted%) [a]: 18,898 (71.1)	5–9 n (Weighted%) [a]: 4849 (17.8)	Total n (Weighted%) [a]: 26,691 (100)
Age (in Years)				
Mean (95% CI)	51.6 (50.6, 52.5)	47.7 (47.3, 48.0)	48.4 (47.8, 49.1)	48.2 (47.9, 48.5)
Sex				
Female	1389 (42.8)	10,110 (50.2)	3052 (61.4)	14,551 (51.4)
Male	1554 (57.2)	8787 (49.8)	1796 (38.6)	12,137 (48.6)
Race and ethnicity				
Hispanic	626 (26.6)	2575 (13.3)	589 (14.5)	3790 (17.1)
Non-Hispanic Asian	297 (10.5)	1161 (6.1)	150 (3.0)	1608 (6.0)
Non-Hispanic Black	409 (13.9)	2056 (11.6)	452 (10.2)	2917 (11.6)
Non-Hispanic Other [b]	71 (2.8)	433 (2.5)	158 (3.8)	662 (2.8)
Non-Hispanic White	1541 (46.2)	12,673 (63.4)	3500 (68.8)	17,714 (62.5)
Education				
Less than high school	420 (18.2)	1376 (9.4)	446 (10.8)	2242 (10.6)
HS graduate/GED	880 (31.7)	4502 (25.7)	1308 (29.4)	6690 (27.0)
Some college	395 (14.3)	2713 (15.9)	855 (19.0)	3963 (16.3)
Associate	343 (11.7)	2500 (13.3)	679 (14.0)	3522 (13.2)
Bachelor	530 (15.1)	4641 (22.0)	949 (17.1)	6120 (20.3)
Graduate degree	356 (9.1)	3084 (13.8)	583 (9.7)	4023 (12.6)
Ratio family income to poverty threshold [c]				
<1 (below poverty level)	368 (12.4)	1582 (8.3)	692 (12.7)	2780 (9.5)
1	604 (21.7)	3055 (16.4)	993 (20.4)	4839 (17.7)
2	488 (117.3)	2793 (15.1)	872 (19.5)	4313 (16.1)
3	403 (114.1)	2538 (12.9)	609 (12.7)	3680 (13.0)
4	292 (9.4)	2221 (12.0)	469 (9.8)	3071 (11.3)
≥5	789 (25.0)	6709 (35.3)	1214 (24.9)	8968 (32.3)

Table 1. Cont.

Characteristics	Insomnia Symptom Scores			
	0 n (Weighted%) [a]: 2944 (11.1)	1–4 n (Weighted%) [a]: 18,898 (71.1)	5–9 n (Weighted%) [a]: 4849 (17.8)	Total n (Weighted%) [a]: 26,691 (100)
Marital status				
Married	1407 (53.6)	8918 (52.7)	1920 (45.9)	12,245 (51.6)
In couple	144 (6.8)	1243 (8.8)	371 (10.5)	1758 (8.9)
Neither	1346 (39.6)	8528 (38.4)	2503 (43.6)	12,377 (39.5)
Smoking status				
Current	314 (10.7)	1924 (10.1)	855 (17.6)	3093 (11.5)
Former	698 (21.4)	4563 (21.4)	1420 (27.0)	6681 (22.4)
Never	1928 (67.8)	12,378 (68.5)	2566 (55.4)	16,872 (66.1)
Alcohol consumption				
Abstainer	652 (24.5)	2102 (12.9)	385 (8.8)	3139 (13.4)
Former	643 (20.5)	3327 (15.7)	1115 (21.1)	5085 (17.2)
Current	1637 (55.0)	13,386 (71.4)	3332 (70.1)	18,355 (69.4)
Physical activity				
Inactive	859 (30.2)	4657 (24.4)	1781 (36.2)	7297 (27.2)
Insufficiently active	654 (21.9)	4939 (26.1)	1237 (25.6)	6830 (25.5)
Sufficiently active	1385 (47.9)	9120 (49.5)	1791 (38.2)	12,296 (47.3)
BMI Group				
Underweight (BMI ≤ 18.4)	46 (1.6)	295 (1.7)	72 (1.8)	413 (1.7)
Healthy weight (18.5–24.9)	1001 (35.0)	5961 (32.0)	1254 (26.5)	8216 (31.3)
Overweight (25–29.9)	1072 (37.1)	6375 (34.0)	1521 (30.9)	8968 (33.8)
Obese (BMI ≥ 30)	745 (26.4)	5894 (32.4)	1892 (40.8)	8531 (33.2)
Sleeping pills				
Never	2749 (94.3)	15,599 (84.0)	2820 (60.0)	21,218 (80.9)
Some days	48 (1.6)	1817 (9.1)	777 (15.8)	2646 (9.5)
Most days	13 (0.4)	311 (1.5)	278 (5.7)	602 (2.1)
Every day	134 (3.6)	1169 (5.4)	970 (18.5)	2280 (7.5)
Diabetes				
Yes	278 (8.5)	1842 (8.7)	716 (13.5)	2836 (9.6)
Hypertension				
Yes	1019 (30.0)	6673 (30.5)	2113 (39.4)	9805 (32.0)
Elevated cholesterol				
Yes	810 (24.0)	5808 (26.4)	1832 (33.3)	8450 (27.4)
Heart disease [d]				
Yes	207 (5.6)	1381 (5.8)	569 (10.0)	2157 (6.5)
Stroke				
Yes	123 (3.5)	581 (2.3)	255 (4.3)	959 (2.8)
Cancer				
Yes	304 (7.8)	2294 (9.1)	738 (12.8)	3336 (9.6)

[a] weighted to account for complex sampling design; [b] other single and multiple races; [c] ratio of family income to poverty threshold for sample adult's family; [d] coronary heart disease, angina, heart attack. Data Source: National Center for Health Statistics, National Health Interview Survey, 2022.

3.2. Association Between Insomnia Symptom Scores and Mental Health

After adjusting for all the covariates, the association between insomnia symptoms and mental health outcomes remained significant (Table 2). Every one-unit increase in insomnia symptom scores was associated with 34% increased odds of anxiety for females (OR = 1.34; 95% CI = 1.31, 1.38) and 38% for males (OR = 1.38; 94% CI: 1.33, 1.42). Similarly, insomnia symptoms were associated with depression for both females (OR = 1.38; 95% CI: 1.34, 1.41) and males (OR = 1.40; 95% CI: 1.36, 1.44). The association was slightly higher for males than for females. A clear dose-response was observed between insomnia symptoms and mental health; as insomnia symptom scores increased, the odds of anxiety and depression also increased in both females and males (Figure 1).

Table 2. Association between insomnia symptom scores and mental health (1 unit increase in insomnia score).

	Crude	Adjusted
	Females	
Anxiety		
All	1.39 (1.36, 1.43)	1.28 (1.24, 1.31)
Age < 50	1.45 (1.40, 1.50)	1.34 (1.29, 1.40)
Age ≥ 50	1.35 (1.31, 1.39)	1.20 (1.16, 1.24)
Depression		
All	1.44 (1.41, 1.47)	1.31 (1.28, 1.35)
Age < 50	1.51 (1.46, 1.57)	1.40 (1.35, 1.46)
Age ≥ 50	1.37 (1.33, 1.41)	1.22 (1.18, 1.26)
	Males	
Anxiety		
All	1.42 (1.38, 1.46)	1.30 (1.26, 1.34)
Age < 50	1.48 (1.42, 1.55)	1.37 (1.30, 1.43)
Age ≥ 50	1.36 (1.31, 1.41)	1.22 (1.17, 1.28)
Depression		
All	1.46 (1.41, 1.50)	1.33 (1.28, 1.37)
Age < 50	1.51 (1.44, 1.57)	1.37 (1.31, 1.44)
Age ≥ 50	1.41 (1.35, 1.47)	1.27 (1.21, 1.33)

Adjusted for age, race and ethnicity, education level, marital status, ratio of family income to poverty threshold, smoking, alcohol consumption, physical activity, body mass index, diabetes, hypertension, heart disease, stroke, cancer, and sleeping pill utilization. Data Source: National Center for Health Statistics, National Health Interview Survey, 2022.

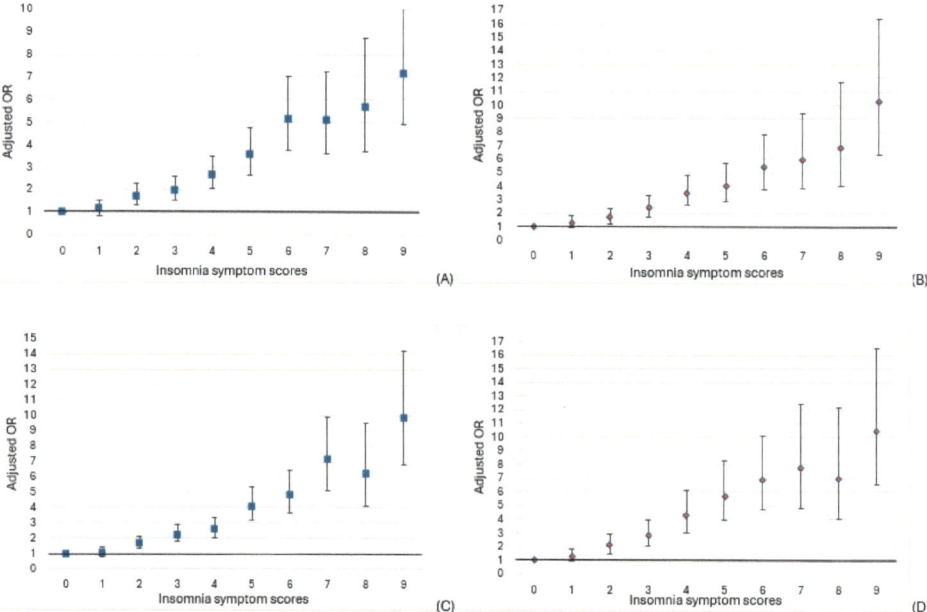

Figure 1. Association between insomnia symptom scores and (**A**) anxiety in females, (**B**) anxiety in males, (**C**) depression in females, and (**D**) depression in males.

The association between insomnia symptoms and mental health outcomes was different by age in both males and females (Table 2). The association was stronger in younger (<50 years) than older adults (≥50 years). For example, females aged <50 years had substantially higher odds of anxiety (OR: 1.34; 95%: 1.29, 1.40) compared to females aged ≥50 years (OR: 1.20; 95% CI: 1.29, 1.40). This pattern was consistent for anxiety and depression in both males and females. However, there was no difference by race and ethnicity, or place of residence (metropolitan or nonmetropolitan). In the individual insomnia symptoms analysis, all three symptoms (difficulty initiating sleep, difficulty maintaining sleep, and non-restorative sleep) were associated with anxiety and depression.

3.3. Mental Health Care Utilization and Barriers in Those with Insomnia Symptoms

After adjusting for all covariates, there was a slight increase in the odds ratios compared to the unadjusted model (Table 3), with females with insomnia symptoms having almost 2 times the odds of receiving mental health care in the past year (OR = 1.7; 95% CI = 1.53, 1.87), delaying mental health care because of its cost (OR = 1.96; 95% CI: 1.67, 2.30), and needing mental health care but not getting it because of the cost (OR = 2.14; 95% CI: 1.82, 2.50) than their males counterpart.

Table 3. Mental health care utilization and perceived barriers in females vs. males among those with insomnia symptoms.

	Crude	Adjusted
Received mental health care in the past year	1.58 (1.43, 1.73)	1.70 (1.53, 1.87)
Delayed mental health care because of cost	1.85 (1.60, 2.15)	1.96 (1.67, 2.30)
Needed mental health care but did not get it because of the cost	1.97 (1.70, 2.28)	2.14 (1.82, 2.50)

Adjusted for age, race and ethnicity, education level, marital status, ratio of family income to poverty threshold, smoking, alcohol consumption, physical activity, body mass index, diabetes, hypertension, heart disease, stroke, and cancer. Data Source: National Center for Health Statistics, National Health Interview Survey, 2022.

Insurance coverage and place of residence (metropolitan or nonmetropolitan) were further assessed for moderation and mediation. While there was no evidence of moderation, a significant albeit minimal mediation by insurance coverage and place of residence was observed (Table 4).

Table 4. Mediation and moderation of mental health care utilization and perceived barriers.

	Natural Indirect Effect (OR, 95% CI)	% Mediated (%, 95% CI)	p-Value Interaction
Received mental health care in the past year			
Insurance coverage	1.01 (1.01, 1.02)	2.08 (1.40, 3.02)	0.3145
Residence (metropolitan and nonmetropolitan)	1.00 (1.00, 1.01)	0.72 (0.12, 1.55)	0.3700
Delayed mental health care because of its cost			
Insurance coverage	0.98 (0.97, 0.99)	−3.70 (−6.42, −2.08)	0.4278
Residence (metropolitan and nonmetropolitan)	1.00 (1.00, 1.01)	0.42 (0.04, 1.16)	0.3891
Needed mental health care but did not get it because of the cost			
Insurance coverage	0.98 (0.97, 0.99)	−3.17 (−5.23, −1.83)	0.5826
Residence (metropolitan and nonmetropolitan)	1.00 (1.00, 1.01)	0.49 (0.04, 1.14)	0.8464

Adjusted for age, race and ethnicity, education level, marital status, ratio of family income to poverty threshold, smoking, alcohol consumption, physical activity, body mass index, diabetes, hypertension, heart disease, stroke, and cancer. Data Source: National Center for Health Statistics, National Health Interview Survey, 2022.

4. Discussion

In this study, we found that insomnia symptoms were associated with anxiety and depression in both females and males. The association was slightly stronger in males than in females and more substantial in younger adults than older adults. Females with insomnia symptoms were more likely to have received mental health care in the past year and more likely to experience financial barriers to mental health care than males. These differences in mental health utilization and perceived barriers were partially mediated by insurance coverage and place of residence.

The findings were consistent with previous studies that linked insomnia symptoms to anxiety and depression [10–13]. Similar to our study, Jaussent et al. utilized self-reported insomnia symptoms, but their study was longitudinal and included older adults from France [10]. Neckelmann et al. included a population from Norway with an age distribution comparable to our sample and also used self-reported insomnia symptoms [11]. Both studies reported that insomnia symptoms were associated with anxiety and depression. Our findings contribute to the existing literature by supporting a dose–response relationship in which the likelihood of depression and anxiety increases with higher levels of insomnia. Although the sex difference in the association between insomnia symptoms and mental health was not substantial, males had slightly higher odds of anxiety and depression associated with insomnia symptoms than females. A female's lifespan is marked by experiences and challenges beginning from adolescence, biological changes, gender roles, hormonal changes, childbirth and child rearing, and menopause, with all carrying potential risks of insomnia. As such, females may cope better with insomnia than males, as they may experience insomnia at an earlier age than males or throughout their lifespan, and may develop better resilience or mental health-seeking behavior [21]. In addition, studies support that males self-report mental health and insomnia issues less frequently than females [22]. Moreover, males may experience greater societal pressure and expectations, which could limit opportunities to develop social connections [23]. Social support and networks have been shown to contribute positively to mental health and well-being [24]. Our finding underscores the importance of more awareness around insomnia and mental health, regardless of sex.

Age differences in the association between insomnia symptoms and mental health were substantial, indicating higher odds for younger adults compared to older adults in both males and females. This finding, coupled with the lower mean age in those with insomnia symptoms, suggests that the burden of insomnia is not only higher in younger adults but also more linked to poor mental health. This is particularly alarming given that younger adults make up the core of the workforce essential to maintaining and advancing societal needs. Efforts to reduce stress and burnout and improve work–life balance would likely contribute to a better quality of life and well-being.

In those with insomnia symptoms, females were more likely to receive mental health care, but also more likely to delay mental health care due to financial barriers than males. The reasons that females exhibit higher levels of mental health-seeking behavior compared to their male counterparts may rely on their attentiveness to their internal psychological experiences compared to males. Societal and cultural expectations of hypermasculinity may prevent males from expressing their emotions and seeking help, especially about mental health, as they risk being perceived as weak. Sigma related to mental health, shame, doubts about the effectiveness of mental health care, costs, and other barriers are still prominent [25]. Reducing those barriers and improving mental health care access is paramount to a better society, given the high prevalence of mental health disorders.

Females were about two times more likely to experience financial barriers to mental health care than males. In the U.S., females may have lower financial earnings and resources compared to males, which could play a critical role in limiting access to health care [26]. Reducing income gap disparities will likely contribute to improving access to mental health care. Alternatively, females may encounter more barriers, possibly because their greater awareness of mental health issues and higher likelihood of seeking care make such challenges more apparent compared to males.

We further observed that the female–male differences in mental health care utilization and perceived barriers were only minimally explained by health insurance coverage and area of residence. Additional barriers such as stigma, cultural attitudes, negative perception of treatment, minimization of insomnia symptoms, provider accessibility, or availability could not be assessed in the present study and should be considered in future research.

Our findings further underscore the benefits of making sure insomnia assessments are not overlooked, with diagnoses slipping through the cracks leading to significantly negative health outcomes. Beyond mental health, insomnia has been linked to multiple other chronic diseases, such as cancer, stroke, heart failure, and hypertension [27–30]. The benefits of interrupting insomnia symptoms early in the disease progression cannot be understated, whether by prevention or intervention. By making an appropriate diagnosis of insomnia, there is a chance of targeted clinical intervention, including cognitive behavioral therapy, instead of hoping that insomnia will resolve spontaneously.

Several limitations should be considered when interpreting these findings. This was a cross-sectional study, which limits our ability to determine directionality and establish causal inference. Insomnia symptoms and mental health outcomes were assessed concurrently, and it is unclear which preceded the other. Future studies with longitudinal data are needed to confirm those findings. Furthermore, the survey was based on self-reported data, which are subject to misclassification bias of both the exposure and the outcome. Future studies and data collection should consider including more objective measurements of sleep and mental health. Insomnia symptoms were compiled into a symptom index, which assumed that all symptoms have equal health implications. An analysis by type of insomnia symptom indicated higher odds for trouble initiating sleep compared to trouble maintaining sleep and non-restorative sleep. However, all three individual insomnia symptoms included in the composite score were strongly associated with anxiety and depression. In addition, insomnia symptoms, rather than diagnosed insomnia, were assessed. This research is an observational study and should be interpreted in light of the potential for residual or unmeasured confounding that may influence the observed associations. Lastly, this study focuses solely on the U.S. adult population, and its findings may not be generalizable to other populations with different health care systems and cultural contexts.

Despite these limitations, the NHIS is a large sample, and the design allows for making inferences about the U.S. adult population. This study was innovative in highlighting age and sex differences in the association between insomnia symptoms and further shedding light on mental health care utilization and barriers. These findings have significant implications for public health, policy, health care, and future research. Public health interventions could include raising awareness about insomnia symptoms and mental health, and improving access to mental health care. Policies aimed at improving access to mental health care could include expanding insurance coverage to encompass cognitive behavioral therapy, as well as extending overall health insurance coverage. Mental health counseling and therapy involve diverse professionals, such as psychiatrists, psychologists, primary care providers, nurses, and clinical social workers, who could all benefit from interprofessional collaboration. In rural areas, for example, where specialist availability is scarce, it often rests on the primary care provider to provide a range of care, including mental health care.

5. Conclusions

The association between insomnia symptoms and increased odds of anxiety and depression in both females and males suggests that insomnia symptoms may be an indicator of mental health outcomes regardless of sex. Insomnia symptoms are more strongly associated with mental health in younger adults compared to older adults. Public health interventions should consider targeting younger adults. The study also revealed that females with insomnia symptoms have higher odds of receiving mental health care, but are also more likely to delay treatment due to costs compared to their male counterparts. This underscores the importance of addressing the gender financial gap to ensure affordable mental health care options for females and improving mental health-seeking behaviors for males. Holistic approaches, including prevention, destigmatization, identification, normalizing help seeking, and improving access to mental health care, are warranted.

Author Contributions: Conceptualization, W.S. and A.N.; methodology, W.S.; software, W.S.; validation, W.S., A.N., and J.J.; formal analysis, W.S.; data curation, W.S.; writing—original draft preparation, W.S., J.J., and A.N.; writing—review and editing, A.N., W.S., and J.J.; visualization, W.S., project administration, A.N. All authors have read and agreed to the published version of the manuscript.

Funding: This research received no external funding.

Institutional Review Board Statement: The IRB of the author's institution has determined that IRB review is not required because the data is deidentified and publicly available.

Informed Consent Statement: The informed consent is not required because the data is deidentified and publicly available.

Data Availability Statement: The data used for this analysis are publicly available at https://www.cdc.gov/nchs/nhis/index.html (accessed on 8 January 2025).

Conflicts of Interest: The authors declare no conflicts of interest.

References

1. Substance Abuse and Mental Health Services Administration (SAMHSA). *Key Substance Use and Mental Health Indicators in the United States: Results from the 2018 National Survey on Drug Use and Health*; HHS Publication No. PEP19-5068, NSDUH Series H-54; Center for Behavioral Health Statistics and Quality, Substance Abuse and Mental Health Services Administration: Rockville, MD, USA, 2019.
2. US National Health Statistics Reports, Number 213, 4 November 2024. Available online: https://www.cdc.gov/nchs/data/nhsr/nhsr213.pdf (accessed on 2 February 2025).
3. Brower, K.J. Professional Stigma of Mental Health Issues: Physicians Are Both the Cause and Solution. *Acad. Med.* **2021**, *96*, 635–640. [CrossRef] [PubMed]
4. Wies, B.; Landers, C.; Ienca, M. Digital Mental Health for Young People: A Scoping Review of Ethical Promises and Challenges. *Front. Digit. Health* **2021**, *3*, 697072. [CrossRef] [PubMed]
5. Zhou, L.; Kong, J.; Li, X.; Ren, Q. Sex differences in the effects of sleep disorders on cognitive dysfunction. *Neurosci. Biobehav. Rev.* **2023**, *146*, 105067. [CrossRef] [PubMed]
6. American Psychiatric Association. *Diagnostic and Statistical Manual of Mental Disorders: DSM-5*; American Psychiatric Association: Washington, DC, USA, 2013. [CrossRef]
7. Morin, C.M.; Jarrin, D.C. Epidemiology of Insomnia: Prevalence, Course, Risk Factors, and Public Health Burden. *Sleep Med. Clin.* **2022**, *17*, 173–191. [CrossRef]
8. Vargas, I.; Perlis, M.L. Insomnia and depression: Clinical associations and possible mechanistic links. *Curr. Opin. Psychol.* **2020**, *34*, 95–99. [CrossRef]
9. Sivertsen, B.; Krokstad, S.; Øverland, S.; Mykletun, A. The epidemiology of insomnia: Associations with physical and mental health: The HUNT-2 study. *J. Psychosom. Res.* **2009**, *67*, 109–116. [CrossRef]
10. Jaussent, I.; Bouyer, J.; Ancelin, M.L.; Akbaraly, T.; Peres, K.; Ritchie, K.; Besset, A.; Dauvilliers, Y. Insomnia and daytime sleepiness are risk factors for depressive symptoms in the elderly. *Sleep* **2011**, *8*, 1103–1110. [CrossRef]
11. Neckelmann, D.; Mykletun, A.; Dahl, A.A. Chronic insomnia as a risk factor for developing anxiety and depression. *Sleep* **2007**, *30*, 873–880. [CrossRef]

12. Hertenstein, E.; Feige, B.; Gmeiner, T.; Kienzler, C.; Spiegelhalder, K.; Johann, A.; Baglioni, C. Insomnia as a predictor of mental disorders: A systematic review and meta-analysis. *Sleep Med. Rev.* **2019**, *43*, 9–105. [CrossRef]
13. Li, L.; Wu, C.; Gan, Y.; Qu, X.; Lu, Z. Insomnia and the risk of depression: A meta-analysis of prospective cohort studies. *BMC Psychiatry* **2016**, *16*, 375. [CrossRef]
14. Zeng, L.N.; Zong, Q.Q.; Yang, Y.; Zhang, L.; Xiang, Y.-F.; Ng, C.H.; Chen, L.-G.; Xiang, Y.-T. Gender Difference in the Prevalence of Insomnia: A Meta-Analysis of Observational Studies. *Front. Psychiatry* **2020**, *11*, 577429. [CrossRef] [PubMed]
15. Marver, J.E.; McGlinchey, E.A. Sex differences in insomnia and risk for psychopathology in adolescence. *Curr. Opin. Psychol.* **2020**, *34*, 63–67. [CrossRef] [PubMed]
16. Sialino, L.D.; van Oostrom, S.H.; Wijnhoven, H.A.H.; Picavet, S.; Verschuren, W.M.M.; Visser, M.; Schaap, L.A. Sex differences in mental health among older adults: Investigating time trends and possible risk groups with regard to age, educational level and ethnicity. *Aging Ment. Health* **2021**, *25*, 2355–2364. [CrossRef]
17. Van Droogenbroeck, F.; Spruyt, B.; Keppens, G. Gender differences in mental health problems among adolescents and the role of social support: Results from the Belgian health interview surveys 2008 and 2013. *BMC Psychiatry* **2018**, *18*, 6. [CrossRef]
18. Lord, C.; Sekerovic, Z.; Carrier, J. Sleep regulation and sex hormones exposure in men and women across adulthood. *Pathol. Biol.* **2014**, *62*, 302–310. [CrossRef]
19. National Center for Health Statistics. National Health Interview Survey, 2022 Survey Description. 2023. Available online: https://ftp.cdc.gov/pub/Health_Statistics/NCHS/Dataset_Documentation/NHIS/2022/srvydesc-508.pdf (accessed on 2 February 2025).
20. VanderWeele, T.J. Mediation Analysis: A Practitioner's Guide. *Annu. Rev. Public Health* **2016**, *37*, 17–32. [CrossRef]
21. Zhang, J.; Chan, N.Y.; Lam, S.P.; Li, S.X.; Liu, Y.; Chan, J.W.; Kong, A.P.S.; Ma, R.C.; Chan, K.C.; Li, A.M.; et al. Emergence of sex differences in insomnia symptoms in adolescents: A large-scale school-based study. *Sleep* **2016**, *39*, 1563–1570. [CrossRef]
22. Shi, P.; Yang, A.; Zhao, Q.; Chen, Z.; Ren, X.; Dai, Q. A Hypothesis of Gender Differences in Self-Reporting Symptom of Depression: Implications to Solve Under-Diagnosis and Under-Treatment of Depression in Males. *Front. Psychiatry* **2021**, *12*, 589687. [CrossRef]
23. Good, G.E.; Sherrod, N.B. The psychology of men and masculinity: Research status and future directions. In *Handbook of the Psychology of Women and Gender*; John Wiley & Sons, Inc.: Hoboken, NJ, USA, 2001.
24. Weitzel, E.C.; Glaesmer, H.; Hinz, A.; Zeynalova, S.; Henger, S.; Engel, C.; Löffler, M.; Reyes, N.; Wirkner, K.; Witte, A.V.; et al. What Builds Resilience? Sociodemographic and Social Correlates in the Population-Based LIFE-Adult-Study. *Int. J. Environ. Res. Public Health* **2022**, *19*, 9601. [CrossRef]
25. Carbonell, Á.; Navarro-Pérez, J.J.; Mestre, M.V. Challenges and barriers in mental healthcare systems and their impact on the family: A systematic integrative review. *Health Soc. Care Community* **2020**, *28*, 1366–1379. [CrossRef]
26. Binder, A.J.; Eng, A.; Houghton, K.; Foote, A. The Gender Pay Gap and Its Determinants Across the Human Capital Distribution; US Census Bureau, Center for Economic Studies: 2024. Available online: www.census.gov/ces (accessed on 18 April 2025).
27. Yoon, K.; Shin, C.M.; Han, K.; Jung, J.H.; Jin, E.H.; Lim, J.H.; Kang, S.J.; Choi, Y.J.; Lee, D.H. Risk of cancer in patients with insomnia: Nationwide retrospective cohort study (2009–2018). *PLoS ONE* **2023**, *18*, e0284494. [CrossRef] [PubMed]
28. Sawadogo, W.; Adera, T.; Alattar, M.; Perera, R.; Burch, J.B. Association Between Insomnia Symptoms and Trajectory with the Risk of Stroke in the Health and Retirement Study. *Neurology* **2023**, *101*, E475–E488. [CrossRef] [PubMed]
29. Mahmood, A.; Ray, M.; Dobalian, A.; Ward, K.D.; Ahn, S.N. Insomnia symptoms and incident heart failure: A population-based cohort study. *Eur. Heart J.* **2021**, *42*, 4169–4176. [CrossRef]
30. Li, L.; Gan, Y.; Zhou, X.; Jiang, H.; Zhao, Y.; Tian, Q.; He, Y.; Liu, Q.; Mei, Q.; Wu, C. Insomnia and the risk of hypertension: A meta-analysis of prospective cohort studies. *Sleep Med. Rev.* **2021**, *56*, 101403. [CrossRef]

Disclaimer/Publisher's Note: The statements, opinions and data contained in all publications are solely those of the individual author(s) and contributor(s) and not of MDPI and/or the editor(s). MDPI and/or the editor(s) disclaim responsibility for any injury to people or property resulting from any ideas, methods, instructions or products referred to in the content.

MDPI AG
Grosspeteranlage 5
4052 Basel
Switzerland
Tel.: +41 61 683 77 34

Journal of Clinical Medicine Editorial Office
E-mail: jcm@mdpi.com
www.mdpi.com/journal/jcm

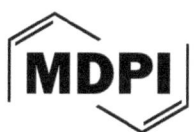

Disclaimer/Publisher's Note: The title and front matter of this reprint are at the discretion of the Guest Editor. The publisher is not responsible for their content or any associated concerns. The statements, opinions and data contained in all individual articles are solely those of the individual Editor and contributors and not of MDPI. MDPI disclaims responsibility for any injury to people or property resulting from any ideas, methods, instructions or products referred to in the content.

www.ingramcontent.com/pod-product-compliance
Lightning Source LLC
LaVergne TN
LVHW070001100526
838202LV00019B/2605